a deeper appreciation and understanding of the broad range of behaviors and value systems I encounter through my work in public education.

Don Hamby
Superintendent of Schools
Willow Springs Public Schools

W9-CFK-289

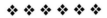

After just 4 days of PeopleWise brain technology training, I increased my free throw shooting to above 90 percent and retained this level of performance in both game and practice for the rest of my playing career. As a head coach, I use PeopleWise to help individual players improve their basketball skills as well as motivate them to work as a team.

Rod Barnes
Head Basketball Coach
The University of Mississippi

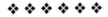

Three years ago our entire maintenance staff completed PeopleWise training. We not only learned how to deal with our differences, but we also learned how to appreciate differences in people. We got immediate results and from time to time various staff members refer back to ideas and concepts learned during the training. PeopleWise is effective, both short-term and long-range.

Fred Davis
Executive Director of Facilities & Operations
Jackson Public Schools

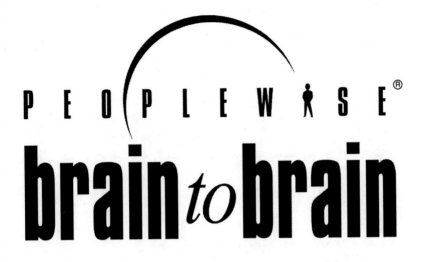

PEOPLEWISE®
brain *to* brain

Dr. James Payne

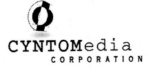

CYNTOMedia
CORPORATION

Pittsburgh, PA

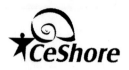

ISBN 1-58501-081-2

Paperback Fiction
© Copyright 2004 Dr. James Payne
All rights reserved
First Printing—2004
Library of Congress #2004106634

Request for information should be addressed to:

SterlingHouse Publisher, Inc.
7436 Washington Avenue
Pittsburgh, PA 15218
www.sterlinghousepublisher.com

CeShore is an imprint of SterlingHouse Publisher, Inc.

SterlingHouse Publisher, Inc. is a company of the CyntoMedia Corporation

Art Director: Matthew J. Lorenz
Cover Design: Matthew J. Lorenz - SterlingHouse Publisher
Typesetting & Layout Design: N. J. McBeth
Illustration/Cover Art: Matthew J. Lorenz

This publication includes images from Corel Draw 8 which are protected
by the copyright laws of the US, Canada, and elsewhere

This is a work of fiction. Names, characters, incidents, and places, are the
product of the author's imagination or are used fictitiously. Any resemblance
to actual events or persons, living or dead is entirely coincidental.

Printed in the United States of America

Dedicated to

Mrs. Margaret McCausland

formerly

Ol' Miss Southworth

A master motivator and

most PeopleWise person

I have ever known.

ACKNOWLEDGMENTS

This work could not have been possible without the active involvement of many university students, close friends, helpful associates, and individual clients representing business, industry, sports, education, vocational rehabilitation, mental health, social services, and the military. The text presents an abundance of actual cases, anecdotes, and stories. To protect the confidentiality of individuals and organizations, names have been changed where appropriate.

PeopleWise® evolved over a period of 30 years and the number of individuals who contributed, directly and indirectly, are too numerous to list. However, special acknowledgment goes to:

Esim Payne, my wife, who encouraged me to continue when I academically stumbled, and, through her mastery of the English language, kept forcing me to clarify paragraph upon paragraph.

Jennifer Piemme, my agent, who saw a bit of talent in me after rejection, after rejection, after rejection.

Cindy Sterling, my publisher, who assembled a team of talented individuals who put PeopleWise® on the market.

Melissa Hudak, production manager, who kept everything rolling and whose creative talents are expressed in the creation of the cover and throughout the format of the book.

Jennifer Bielata, proof reader and editor, who helped make the book flow and be reader-friendly.

And lastly,

Shirley Messer, typist, friend, and confidant, who kept typing and retyping the manuscript year after year without complaint.

PREFACE

The world would be sad and silent
if no birds sang except the very best.

– Anonymous

Within you lies a song not sung, a sound not heard, an action not taken, a life yet to throb to a swifter beat. The danger in life is not failure, the danger in life is that dreaded nothingness. If you haven't failed, you haven't tried, and until you try, you can't succeed. The secret to success lies within your mind and the secret to understanding the mind lies within this book.

The eminent philosopher, William James, coined the term "over beliefs." Over beliefs are known facts that the facts themselves do not justify. As a practical measure, these over beliefs are not only permissible but also, according to James, they are necessary. Our assumption of a projected idea, goal, and/or happening which we cannot, at that moment, see is what dictates our present actions and our practical conduct. In other words, PeopleWise® Motivation is an over belief that takes a series of facts on motivation and extrapolates them into a usable application that helps us immediately improve ourselves.

Thanks to computerized electrodes that measure the activation of the brain, you can, with minimal training, control your own thought waves and place success in the center of your life. This powerful, dynamic, mental artistry, when applied systematically and conscientiously, produces three major benefits. These are self-motivation which provides complete self-empowerment, expanded interpersonal relationships with others, and improved physical skill development. Once understood, the complexity and dynamics of this brain technology can be learned and taught by anyone, at any time, in any place — without any equipment.

The reason personal brain control is not public knowledge is because three separate disciplines each hold a vital piece to the brain technology puzzle. These disciplines refuse to share their expertise with individuals outside of their own fields. These three areas of expertise are: personal development, sometimes referred to as visual imagery; the area of personality differences, sometimes referred to as learning styles or management types; and lastly, the discipline of brain technology, which deals with the firing of the brain. PeopleWise® Motivation takes information from each of these three areas and combines them into an understandable and powerful system of self improvement.

PEOPLEWISE® MOTIVATION: The Art of Motivating Brain-to-Brain helps you understand the connection between how people behave and the activation of the brain. As you learn how the functioning of the brain affects how people react and respond to various situations, you learn how you can improve your own managing, coaching, counseling, teaching, and parenting. You also learn how you can utilize brain technology to improve your own thinking, problem solving, visioning, and your own skill development.

PeopleWise® Motivation will provide you with a huge arsenal of powerful techniques which will dramatically help you attain Olympian confidence and focus that will enhance your concentration and improve your performance. As you master mind-control, you will begin revving up the activation of your mind that will ultimately turbo-charge your performance. PeopleWise® Motivation reveals the complexities of human behavior in usable, understandable terms. The brilliance is in its simplicity. Let me share what I have learned about an advanced understanding of human behavior. Come with me as I unveil this well-kept secret of the mind — **PeopleWise® Motivation.** You will sing like you have never sung before.

J. S. P.

TABLE OF CONTENTS

PART I:
VISUAL IMAGERY
(SELF-MOTIVATION)

CHAPTER ONE

Comfort Zones Know Math

Mary Rodriguez is alone this early morning. She is well into her practice round, preparing for tomorrow's ladies' annual golf tournament. She has been striking the ball solidly. On every hole she has been in the fairway and on the green in regulation. Now she is at the dreaded Number Eight. A seemingly simple, 120 yard par 3. Fifty yards from the tee is a pond that stretches to within 10 yards of the green. For Mary, this is an easy eight iron.

As she approaches the tee, she glances at the pond out of the corner of her eye. She tees up the ball, positions herself, waggles the club, takes one more look at the pin, and then abruptly turns away and walks to her bag. She unzips the top pocket of her bag and takes out a used, scuffed-up ball. She approaches the tee and replaces the new, good ball with the old one.

Now ready, she addresses the ball, glances at the flag, mutters a brief prayer, waggles the club, draws the club back and, right before she starts her down swing, a resounding voice bolts out from the sky: "STOP, BE CONFIDENT, TEE UP A NEW BALL."

Somewhat shaken, she takes the new ball out of her pocket and replaces the used ball. Uneasy but compliant, she glances at the water, addresses the ball, waggles the club, begins to draw the club back and again, booming from the sky: "STOP, STEP BACK AND TAKE A PRACTICE SWING."

Mary, confused but obedient, steps away from the ball, positions herself, and takes a practice swing. She hesitates a moment, then takes a second practice swing, then a third, fourth, and fifth. Now ready, if not over-ready, she steps forward, addresses the ball, begins her swing and, from the sky, in an authoritarian tone: "ON SECOND THOUGHT, TEE UP THE USED BALL."

Just what is confidence? Confidence is knowing you are going to be successful **before** you execute the task regardless of what others may tell you. PeopleWise® is a system that teaches every person how the brain really ticks and what can be done to bolster confidence that will produce self-empowerment.

Homerun champion Mark McGwire, during an October 1998 interview on CNN, was asked: "What are you doing differently now that has made you so great?" His matter-of-fact response was, "Two years ago I learned the importance of the mental part of the game." He was saying that he had learned how to control his focus and his thought processes. You could see it each time he got ready to bat. In the on-deck circle, rather than physically practice swinging, he used this time to mentally prepare himself. That's right, in the on-deck circle, Mark McGwire did **not** physically practice swinging the bat, he used this time to **mentally** prepare himself. On September 27, 1998, Mark McGwire smashed Babe Ruth's and Roger Maris' long-standing homerun records by hitting 70 homeruns.

Before becoming nationally famous, Jim Thorpe, great all-time athlete, is said to have finished his race and immediately reported to the long jump area at Haskell Institute in Lawrence, Kansas. He walked to the landing area and placed his warmup jacket next to the pit. He returned to the approach area, sat in a lotus position with his legs crossed, forearms on his knees, thumbs on each hand pressed against his index finger and his eyes focused on the jacket. After a short time, an official came to Jim Thorpe and asked if he'd like to take a couple of practice jumps. As dictated to me during interviews with admirers of Jim Thorpe, he replied, "I already have, 25 times." Jim Thorpe had already **mentally** successfully jumped 25 times. That day he won the event as he had done so many times before and as he continued to do throughout his life.

On September 15, 2001, during a conversation with Lane Vines, golf pro, Grand Oaks Country Club, Oxford, Mississippi, he reported that one time Lee Trevino, golfing great, studied an eight-foot putt on the last hole. He was with his friends and had a small wager on the side. He needed this putt to win. The ball was struck, a crisp ping resounded through the air, followed by a plop as the ball fell into the bottom of the cup. Lee Trevino smiled, pumped his fists triumphantly into the air, while his opponents shook their heads in disbelief. It's not so spectacular that he made the putt, what made it great is he tapped it in with a Dr. Pepper bottle.

Rumor has it that on many occasions he putted with a Dr. Pepper bottle. Is it any wonder that later in his career, Dr. Pepper became one of his major sponsors?

Confidence can be learned. Confidence can be taught. Confidence is training your "mind's eye" to mentally see the successful outcome before it happens.

The rain is starting to fall this early afternoon of October 1989 in Broken Arrow, Oklahoma. Ruth Brookfield, manager and long-time client, jumps out of her car and runs into Domino's Pizza. She straps on her apron, straightens her cap, checks over the freshly stocked ingredients' table, lays out several trays of dough, turns up the temperature on the ovens, and immediately goes into a trance-like state, much like a Buddha preparing for serious meditation. The rain, coupled with it being a game day, plus America's number one TV program is airing this evening: Ruth Brookfield regains focus as six phones begin to ring and six attendants take orders at lightning speed. This will be a banner evening and everyone knows it. Tonight, Ruth is in her element. She moves with the gracefulness of a ninja warrior and the quickness of a karate expert. Ruth is a one-person whirlwind, preparing each pizza unassisted and shoving them in the ovens. Six hundred and fifty pizzas later, Ruth gives a high five to the phone attendants. The delivery persons are jubilant and the place is rocking with happiness. A personal best is experienced as another record goes into the books.

Every June of every year, my oldest daughter, Kimberly Sue Simmons in Dover, Delaware, prepares for an important awards dinner that is to be held in her home. Weeks of preparation have gone into this event and everything has been double and triple checked. Kimberly and her husband are dressed to the hilt but, before the first guest arrives, Kimberly retreats to the bedroom and now, alone with eyes closed, she mentally imagines each guest having a good time. She mentally plays out all the options she will encounter this evening and how she will respond. As she programs her mind, she experiences what it feels like to be a successful hostess. Needless to say, the evening is spectacular and exceeds everyone's highest expectations.

Every day in the employees' locker room at the IBP meat packing plant in Emporia, Kansas, Maria Sanchez, a valued client of mine, puts on her work clothes and prepares to package meat. Her job is to take meat from a chute and put three pieces in a 8" x 12" plastic bag and then stack the filled bags in boxes to be shipped. Maria Sanchez sacks significantly more than any other employee. She does this every night and she enjoys doing it as much as a professional athlete enjoys performing their job. It is important to note that prior to reporting to her work station on the floor, she visualizes the moves, kinesthetically feels the rhythm necessary to perform the task at record speed, and actually gets excited before sacking her first pieces of meat. Maria Sanchez is world class and everyone at IBP knows it.

Extraordinary performance is recorded in unusual places by ordinary people who are prepared, talented, and confident. Once a person is prepared and they have demonstrated talent for doing the task, what remains is mental. For the skilled and talented, the mental part of superior task execution makes up 90 percent of the total effort involved. For the skilled and talented, this 90 percent often separates the great from the very good, a legend from a top professional, the champion from the runner-up. To realize the value of one milli-second, ask the person who has won a **silver** medal in the Olympics. As one approaches world class, we may be talking millimeters and nanoseconds. For most of us, we are striving for a personal best.

Recently, computerized electrodes have become available that somewhat accurately measure the activation impulses of the brain. These instruments provide information that suggests that in most people, most of the time, the activation activity in the brain is somewhat scattered. However, when a person begins to concentrate or focus on something with a high degree of intensity, the activation of the brain becomes more localized in a specific section of the brain. When the concentration or focus becomes so intense that the individual enters a state of consciousness known as the "zone" or "flow," the activation becomes pinpointed in a relatively small area. It is important to understand that the firing of the brain is more localized when a person is in a high state of concentration, but it is breathtaking to learn that people can actually control the firing of their own brain waves. People can be taught how to control their brain activation. In other words, people can be taught how to improve their concentration and focus. Mastering mind control begins with understanding the comfort zone.

Everyone has a mental picture of who they are and what they can and cannot do. There are success personalities and failure personalities, optimists and pessimists, extroverts and introverts. If a person believes they can't do something, even if it is well within their capacity, then chances are they are not going to do it. If a person believes they can do it and if they have the skill and talent to do it, then it is more than likely they will do it. If a person thinks they can't do it and they actually do it, more times than not the person attributes it to luck, the weather, fate, or chance. When the activity is repeated again, after a successful accomplishment attributed to outside forces, it is likely the individual will fail. The failure validates the individual's picture that they couldn't do it in the first place. The failure reinforces the belief they can't do it.

People behave in accordance with their pictures. People validate their mental pictures time and time again. This mental picture is our comfort zone.

Joan is a graduate student of mine as well as a successful manager at a large department store in Memphis, Tennessee. Every Wednesday night several of the employees compete in a local bowling tournament. Joan is one of the league's top bowlers, carrying an average of 192. Tonight, Joan is on a roll. She is ready to finish the 10th frame with three pins standing. She holds a 218, a personal best. You would think she would be excited and anxious to roll the last ball for a possible 221, but she is nervous, she is fidgety. Her forehead beads with perspiration and her heart is pounding with an unusual thump. She sizes up the pins, begins her approach, releases the ball and knocks down all three for a 221. She jumps up and down, everyone congratulates her. There is a spirit of celebration in the building and the owner issues all of her team a free round of drinks.

Now think what has happened. Joan has demonstrated she can bowl a 221. She has done it, experienced it, and been reinforced for it. So one would think that she would do it again, but you know, I know, and the world knows that during the next line she will not bowl a 221. She won't even bowl her average. She will most likely score significantly below her average. During the next line she actually scores a 169. Why? She pictures herself as a 192 bowler and she bowls around 192, she feels comfortable. Sometimes she will score a little higher and sometimes a little lower, but she always averages 192 no matter how much she practices. All of a sudden she scores a whopping 221. She is excited, happy, even ecstatic, but she is uncomfortable. She has performed outside her comfort zone. A 221 is not normal. It is not her. A 221 is beyond her grasp, beyond her highest expectation. Simply put, the 221 was just plain ol' luck. It just sort of happened. It came out of left field. So the next time she bowls significantly below her average and she says to herself, "I knew it, I'm a 192er."

Everyone has seen this happen or has experienced it themselves, yet no one understands this phenomenon. The answer is, the comfort zone knows math. It can add, subtract, multiply and divide. The comfort zone is what makes us sane, what makes us real, what makes us "us." If Joan continued to bowl 221, she would have gone out of her mind, because she knows deep down inside that 221 is not her; she is a 192er.

As a motivational consultant, I am asked to work with sales departments to improve sales. Typically, I go into an organization, get the sales force excited, get them focused on selling, start some type of competitive contest, recognize outstanding achievement, and sure enough, the sales department will show a significant increase in sales. Why? Simply put, they become motivated to sell. Unfortunately, when I leave, the next month's sales will plummet. Why? They know, as salespersons, who they are. They will function within their picture of who they are and continue to do it, day in and day out, again and again. I enter the picture and they sell more merchandise. This places them outside that picture, outside their comfort zone; thus, when I leave, they will balance it out mathematically. The result is they sell less than they did before I entered the scene. In essence, in a matter of days they return to their average. The comfort zone knows math, but we can outsmart it.

CHAPTER TWO

Outsmarting the Comfort Zone

Martha Parrish is a high school teacher outside of Houston, Texas. She has developed a program where students donate their time giving something back to the community. Several articles have appeared in the newspaper highlighting Martha's class and she is asked to speak at the local Pilot Club. She is a shy, humble person and sees herself as a public servant, not a public speaker. In fact, she believes she can't speak before groups. Her students and the principal pressure her to speak at a November 12th meeting. Hesitant but determined, she outlines her speech, puts her presentation on 3" x 5" note cards and practices in the privacy of her own home. She gets it down perfectly. Her message is clear, substantive, and sprinkled lightly with appropriate humor.

The 12th arrives. She dresses appropriately, everyone is served lunch and, after a little housekeeping, she is introduced by the chairperson. Applause fills the air as she confidently approaches the lectern. She has written the speech, placed the salient points in large type on note cards, and rehearsed it over 100 times. She lays the cards on the lectern and just as she is about to begin, she looks up and, lo and behold, she sees the audience's gaze glued on her. She hesitates and strangely, out of her mouth, in a high-pitched voice, much like that of Alvin and the Chipmunks, she utters, "I am excited to be here to share what our students are doing."

She struggles from card to card. Moisture begins to form above her upper lip, and she experiences small hot flashes from time to time. She finally finishes and returns to her seat at the head table as the audience applauds. She believes they are just being polite because she knows she did a terrible job.

What made her voice become so high pitched? What made her lose her place? What made her sweat? What made her nervous? It is the power of the comfort zone. When we try to function outside our comfort zone, things happen to put us right smack-dab back into the middle of our comfort zone. This is what makes us who we are. This is what makes us normal. This is what makes us sane. This is what makes us "us."

If Martha had, in fact, done a good job of speaking, then she would probably have thought it was just luck or a trick of some sort and next time she would have been awful, if not downright pitiful. A pitiful performance would be necessary to balance out an excellent performance in order for her to validate her picture of not being able to speak before groups. Simply put, her comfort zone was "an inability to speak before groups." She believed this with all her heart and she knew she couldn't do it. So when the time arose to speak, she fouled up, which validated her picture of "I can't speak before groups." Let's face it, Martha can't speak before groups.

Some people believe they can't remember names. They are of normal intelligence and their minds work perfectly, but no matter how much they try, how much they practice, how many memory courses they take, if they believe they can't remember names, then they just flat won't remember names. The comfort zone is so very powerful it locks us into acting and behaving as we see ourselves and believe ourselves to be. We act and behave in accordance with our picture. Our picture is our life's target. Our comfort zone is nothing more than a target of life. What keeps us on target, what keeps us functioning within our comfort zone is the creative subconscious.

Maxwell Maltz, M.D., a famous plastic surgeon and best-selling author of *Psycho-Cybernetics*, suggests the mind (creative subconscious) is like a homing system in a torpedo or an automatic pilot. Once the target is set, the self-adjusting mechanism guides the missile toward the target through a monitoring feedback system. This navigational guidance system constantly adjusts the flight of the missile by keeping it on target. Just as the propulsion of the missile drives it forward, the creative subconscious drives our behavior and actions. In other words, the creative subconscious is our motivator. The creative subconscious motivates us to perform within our comfort zone.

We cannot control the creative subconscious. The creative subconscious is always programmed to guide our behaviors and actions toward our picture, toward our comfort zone, toward our target. But the beauty is we can move our picture, change our comfort zone, select a new target. We can outsmart our comfort zone by talking ourselves into believing we are different. We can tell ourselves over and over again, with such conviction, that we can actually see a new picture of ourselves, vividly, in high resolution. As we construct a new target of ourselves, the creative subconscious will drive us, monitor us, to become it.

It is easy to outsmart the comfort zone because it believes what it hears and feels. Martha Parrish had the skill, talent, and material to be a good speaker. What she didn't have was the confidence or belief she could do it. Her picture of not being able to speak before groups got in her way. To work on the mental part of her game she could have begun to imagine herself speaking successfully before groups. She could tell herself, "I like myself as I present before groups; I see people listening to me with admiration and interest; I see them laughing at my jokes; I see them applauding enthusiastically; I see them giving me a standing ovation; I feel the excitement; I feel joy; I feel the happiness in my heart as I share the students' accomplishments; I feel the pride of having an opportunity to encourage the Pilot Club to assist us with our cause."

By talking to herself in this manner, she could begin to alter her picture of herself as a speaker. She could change her comfort zone, her target. Now, with her new picture, as she prepares she gains confidence because she sees herself successful. She will find she can't wait to present to the Pilot Club because the creative subconscious is driving her toward her new target of being an accomplished speaker.

You have the power to change your target, but you cannot change or control the creative subconscious. The creative subconscious is nothing more than a homing device that drives your behaviors and actions toward the target.

I was asked by the Mississippi State Department of Education to interview successful individuals in Tunica, Mississippi. At the time, Tunica was the poorest county in the continental United States. The purpose of surveying successful individuals of Tunica was to take the information and use it to help the school system to become better and more effective. I talked with proprietors, attorneys, ministers, government officials, and a dentist, but what struck me most was the interview I had with Henry Woodard. Henry was a black man with a second grade education who had scraped and saved to where he owned a good-sized farm. He and his wife raised 17 children, all of whom completed high school, and most went on to attend a nearby community college. I was fascinated by his demeanor and his wisdom. Toward the end of the conference I asked him to share the greatest lesson he had learned. He thought for a minute and replied, "It is hard to go where you have never been — but it can be done when you force yourself to see it."

Outsmarting the comfort zone is nothing more than forcing ourselves to see it. Fortunately, through the works of Maxwell Maltz, Denis Waitley, Louis Tice, and others, we have a program that helps us force ourselves to see ourselves in a different light. As we force ourselves to see it, we develop Mind Control.

I was invited by the governor of Virginia to present to a group of rehabilitation counselors on how to help individuals with severe handicapping conditions to get jobs. The presentation was to be Saturday, 8:30 a.m., in the Coliseum in Virginia Beach. There were to be over 2,000 in attendance and this was a big deal to me. I was leaving from Charlottesville, but I hadn't gotten started as soon as I had hoped. I was traveling east on Highway 64 and was approaching the tunnel that leads into Virginia Beach. It was just past midnight. I was to stay at the Red Roof Inn, located less than a mile from the tunnel. As I emerged from the tunnel I noticed in my rearview mirror two red, flashing, lights. I glanced down to discover I was going 75 miles per hour in a 55 mile per hour zone. I pulled over to the right side of the road, angry at myself, yet simultaneously trying to figure out how I could motivate the officer not to give me a ticket.

Quickly, I thought back to my Boy Scout days — Be Prepared and Anticipate Future Happenings. I realized the officer will ask for my driver's license and car registration. In a flash, I removed my driver's license from my wallet and secured the car registration from the glove box. In an attempt to impress the officer, before anything was said, I handed him my driver's license and car registration. It didn't impress him. He promptly walked back to his vehicle and I could see in my rearview mirror he was writing me a ticket. This made me angry, then I realized, he didn't know who he was dealing with. After all, I was DOCTOR Payne and I was there at the invitation of the GOV-ERNOR, and I was there to help the HANDICAPPED. The officer returned, handed me my driver's license and car registration, explained I was doing 75 in a 55 zone, and then proceeded to instruct me to sign by the X. I tried to explain to him that he didn't fully understand the situation, but he assured me he did. I was doing 75 in a 55. But, I explained, there were some extenuating circumstances. He broke in, explaining this needed to be told to the judge. I cut him off as he was about to tell me my rights, "Look officer, I'm DOCTOR James S. Payne, I'm here at the invitation of the GOVERNOR and tomorrow morning I'm presenting to a group of rehabilitation counselors on how to help the HANDICAPPED. Authoritatively, he rebutted, "DOCTOR Payne, tomorrow, if you want to see the GOVERNOR and help the HANDICAPPED, you better SIGN the ticket or I've got to take you to JAIL." I obediently signed. After signing, he gave me the ticket and promptly walked to his car.

By this time, I was fuming. I thought, why wasn't he out catching real crooks, real burglars, real criminals, why was he messing with me? I waited for him to pull out and realized **he** was waiting for me to pull out first. I put on my blinker, held my arm out the window, hoping this was the proper procedure for pulling out on an interstate. I turned into the entrance to the Red Roof Inn to find no rooms. Since I hadn't confirmed my reservation by 6 p.m., they had released it to another customer. I got so angry, I demanded to see the owner. The owner came out to the office wearing pajamas and listened to my plight. He said there was only one room, but it was under repair. The bed was made, but there was a ladder against the wall and a fresh paint smell. Disgruntled, I took the key, reported to the room, got ready for bed, lay down, to find I couldn't sleep. I got up, turned on the TV, sat on the edge of the bed, and watched for 45 minutes. Suddenly, I realized I didn't even know what I was watching. All I could see was that policeman. I was so upset. I hated policemen. I hated their hats, shirts, badges, boots, and all that stuff they have around their waists. Then it hit me; who was in control of my mind? That policeman was off giving more tickets. He didn't care about me and here I was reacting to him for issuing a ticket. I had allowed that policeman to enter the privacy of my own mind.

How many times do you get out of control? How about when your car won't start, your children unintentionally do something wrong, or things don't go right at work. Many things enter our life and control our thinking. Just as we can alter or change our picture of who we are, we can also control our own thoughts. We may not have control over the situation, but we have 100 percent control over how we respond and react to any given situation.

At that point in time, when I realized I was out of control because the policeman had control of my mind, I went over to the desk in the room, pulled out a piece of stationary, and began to write a couple of things down, which will be explained in detail in Chapter 5. Within less than 5 minutes, I flushed that policeman out of my mind and I took control of my mental processes. I actually wiped my mind clean and began to think positively and creatively. I lay down and slept like a baby. I got up the next morning and gave an excellent presentation and never once thought about the ticket or the policeman again. I had mastered controlling my own mind.

You can do this just as I did and continually do. You will learn to control your own mind. You will be able to activate your brain to such a degree that, if you so choose, you can control your own dreams. You can turn nightmares into pleasant dreams. Mastering mind control can be learned in minutes and applied in seconds. Once mastered it can be used throughout a lifetime.

CHAPTER THREE

MASTERING MIND CONTROL

THE FIRST PART

Just as an Olympian can mentally prepare for a major event, just as a professional salesperson can psych themselves up to become more effective in assisting customers in selecting purchases, just as an executive can prepare for a major meeting, just as an attorney can prepare for a court case, just as a speaker can prepare for a major presentation, just as a hostess can prepare for an important dinner engagement, and just as a child can accelerate their learning through mental discipline, you will be able to control your mind.

There are nine basic steps to mastering mind control.

1. Get a picture of what you want, not what you don't want.

This sounds simple, but you will find it isn't as simple as it appears. Many times we focus on what we don't want rather than what we want. We think about how many pounds we want to lose rather than how much we want to weigh. We think about not slicing the golf ball as opposed to imagining where we want to hit it, right in the middle of the fairway. We focus on not embarrassing ourselves instead of seeing ourselves performing perfectly. We focus on the fact that we don't want to fail instead of identifying success patterns. It is easy, and for some people, very natural to focus on what they don't want rather than what they want.

Louis Tice, renowned motivational expert, refers to this as the "Rock in the Road." He tells the story of learning how to ride a bike. As we begin, it is hard to keep our balance. Soon, we find it is easier to keep the bike balanced if the bike is moving forward; however, because we are unsteady and somewhat unstable, we often find ourselves heading in directions we don't want to go. Many beginning riders find themselves moving forward, only to spot a rock in the road. The more we try to steer away from the rock, the more the rock pulls us toward it. Rather than looking at where we want to go, we look at where we don't want to go — we can't take our eyes off the rock. Tice advises, "Don't lead your people to the rock in the road and don't lead yourself to the rock in the road."

2. Clarify your desire in terms of effort, time, money, risk.

Bringing about a significant change in your life will cost you something. You must be willing to pay the price. Mind control costs. Mind control will take some effort, yet you can't force it. It takes effort and energy. Although initially it won't take a lot of time, later, you might become addicted to the process and find you are practicing mind control many times throughout the day. The monetary cost is usually minimal; however, sometimes aids and self-help devices such as background sound tapes or specific personal development books will be helpful. The real price comes in your willingness to take a risk. You must conquer the fear of failure that so often accompanies risk. One of the best ways to handle fear is to determine what is the worst thing that could happen. In most cases, it isn't severe. We are not talking life or death here. Keep a sense of humor and work at mind control intently, but don't take it too seriously.

3. Fit it into your star-balance.

If you are willing to make the effort and pay the price, then it is important to make sure that what you do is healthy. Make sure it is the right thing for you to do. Make sure it will make you a better person. The key lies in balance. Valiant Thor wrote a rather obscure book, *Outwitting Tomorrow*. The book is small, but it contains the wisdom of volumes. The format of the book centers around two men, Mr. Workman and Mr. Grayson. Mr. Workman is a 65-year-old farmer who chronically bitches and complains. Mr. Grayson is more than 70 years old, but he looks much younger than Workman. The entire book is Grayson teaching Workman about his philosophy of life, a part of which centers around The Five Departments of Life. As Workman learns and practices the philosophy, he grows younger and his rheumatism disappears.

The Five Departments of Life are depicted in the form of a star with each point representing a specific department. Figure 3-1 shows The Departments of Life as (1) Spiritual, (2) Mental, (3) Physical, (4) Social, and (5) Financial. The five departments cover the most important phases of life itself. The sole purpose in life is to fill out all the departments to their fullest. As an individual grows, each department must be evenly and symmetrically filled. If one point is developed beyond other points, the result is a less healthy person, an unbalanced person, or a warped star, so-to-speak.

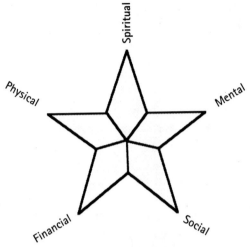

Figure 3-1: Five Departments of Life

As an example, Figure 3-2 represents an over-developed spiritual person. This person is described as "all heart and no head." This person is a narrow thinker, intolerant, and possibly fanatical. This individual has friends of a similar make-up and physically, the person is only a fraction of what the person should be. Over-developed spiritual people are straight-laced and unyielding.

Figure 3-2: Over-Developed Spiritually

As can be anticipated, an over-developed mental person refers to an individual who cares little for physical exercise, thus physical health may be bad; socially, they are confined to associates of similar interests, and they live in a land of theory that is highly impractical. The over-developed physical individual is interested in muscle and body development exclusive of other types of development. An over-developed social person is the outgoing, affable individual. The over-developed financial person is obsessed with money and prestige.

Usually, an individual isn't any one type. Normally people are a combination of types, emphasizing two or three well-developed points. However, most people seem to have one point which is neglected. When an individual has one or more points that are neglected, this retards progress for the development of a complete, fully functioning, healthy individual.

As an individual develops, it is important that The Five Departments of Life are equally, evenly, and steadily developed. As the points of the star fill out, the individual becomes powerful and power-filled. A symmetrical foundation that is solid and strong breeds real and lasting accomplishments. A completely filled star represents an individual who is at harmony with both the visible and unseen worlds and is identified as an all-around person. But this is not the end, for there is no end to psychological development.

Each point on the star is capable of unlimited extension. Figure 3-3 illustrates the elasticity of the star with elongated points. There is no limit to the growth of any department of life. As stated by Valiant Thor in his book *Outwitting Tomorrow*, "when one has experienced thrilling EXPANSION in all Five Departments of Life, there is no turning back. From then on it's a search for 'more worlds to conquer.'" For the expanded person, there are no limits, no sorrows, no darkness. Everyone is a star and capable of doing things that are star-worthy. At this point in mastering mind control, it is important to seriously assess and determine that your imagined target is charted on a healthy path for you and for those you touch.

4. Imagine the end result in vivid detail.

Once you get a picture of what you want and are willing to pay the price and what you decide to undertake is the right thing, then it is important to begin to perfect the image in the most vivid detail possible. The clarity of this picture in the highest resolution is the foundation for real mind control. You must create this picture in such a way that you can see it, hear it, feel it, smell it, and taste it. The clearer and more focused the target, the more efficiently the tracking device of the creative subconscious will work. What motivates a person is not the picture, what motivates the person is the creative subconscious. If the picture is vague, the tracking device doesn't know exactly where to go, so it vacillates all over the place. When the picture is pinpointed, the tracking device is razor sharp.

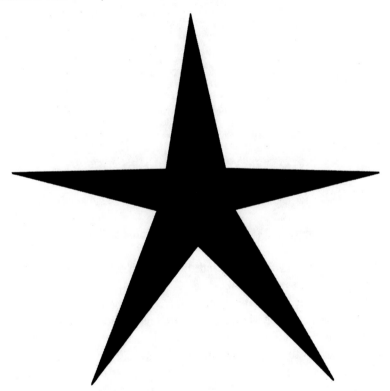

Figure 3-3: The Expanded Person
Even though the subconscious mind cannot distinguish between an imagined picture from the real thing, the subconscious mind also cannot

create a clearer, more vivid picture. Only the conscious mind can craft a vivid image in high resolution. You must now begin to work the conscious part of your mind, realizing your conscious mind has been programmed over time to cope and survive rather than construct and create.

The caption in Figure 3-4 was taken from *Can You Believe Your Eyes?*, a 1988 science article by J. Richard Block and Harold E. Yuker. Read the large-type words in the center of the page, dealing with the problem of AIDS.

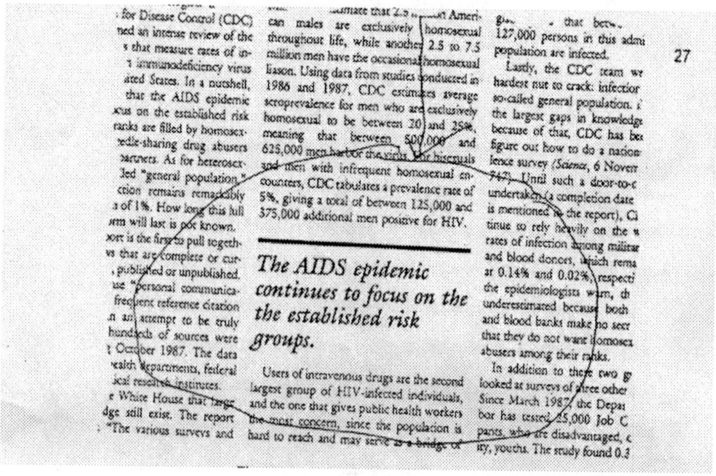

can males are exclusively homosexual throughout life, while another 2.5 to 7.5 million men have the occasional homosexual liaison. Using data from studies conducted in 1986 and 1987, CDC estimates average seroprevalence for men who are exclusively homosexual to be between 20 and 25%, meaning that between 500,000 and 625,000 men ... and men with infrequent homosexual encounters, CDC tabulates a prevalence rate of 5%, giving a total of between 125,000 and 375,000 additional men positive for HIV.

The AIDS epidemic continues to focus on the the established risk groups.

Users of intravenous drugs are the second largest group of HIV-infected individuals, and the one that gives public health workers the most concern, since the population is hard to reach and may serve as a bridge of

Figure 3-4. Taken from the journal Science

Many people, when they read the above, block out the second "the" in ". . . focus on the the established . . . ." This blocking out is referred to as "scotoma." Scotoma means blind spot. Scotoma is a sensory blocking out of external events we have been trained to block out. We go about life forcing ourselves to make sense out of things and to get to the root of things or get to the bottom line. Two "the's" doesn't make sense, so the subconscious blocks out one "the" from the conscious part of the brain so the phrase makes sense. Have you ever tried to find something and it was right in front of you but you couldn't see it? What blocked it out was scotoma. You misplace your keys and your subconscious convinces you that you have lost them. You can be consciously looking straight at your keys but you can't see them. As you begin to imagine the end result in vivid detail, it is imperative you guard yourself from scotoma.

I was working with Hewlett Packard on understanding vision building and they sent me a postcard with a picture on it, as reproduced in Figure 3-5. They asked me to tell them what it was.

Take a look at the picture in Figure 3-5. When I looked at the picture I couldn't figure it out. My staff and I looked at the picture for a couple of weeks and never figured it out. I called the person that sent it to me and he said **turn it around clockwise one-quarter of a turn**. We did and we still couldn't see it. The staff and I looked at it another week. Then, in desperation, we called and pleaded to be told what it was. He said,

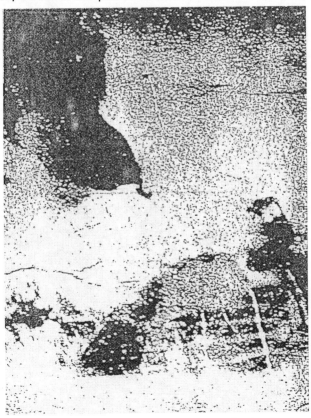

Figure 3-5. Postcard picture from Hewlett Packard

1. It is something very common and it is not hidden. We still couldn't see it. (Do you see it yet?)

2. It is an animal. We still couldn't see it. (Do you see it yet?)

3. It is an animal you see on a farm. We still couldn't see it. (Do you see it yet?)

4. The animal is looking straight at you.

At that moment, Marjorie, the executive secretary, shouted, "I see it, it is a cow." The rest of us looked but still couldn't see it until Marjorie pointed it out to us, at which point we all said, "Oh" because it was so clear. (If you still can't see it, turn to page 203 where it is outlined for you.)

The point of this illustration is that for many people the cow is difficult to see. Yet, once you see it, you can't believe you couldn't see it before. It is so clear. This is similar to what happens when you imagine the end result in vivid detail. In the beginning it is vague, blurry, but as you work on it, it becomes clear and eventually it is very vivid.

As you imagine the end result in vivid detail, guard against scotoma and keep working at it until it becomes crystal clear. It often helps to bring in the other senses, taste, touch, smell. Your imagined "cow" becomes very real in your "mind's eye."

Once we get a picture of what we want without leading ourselves to the rock in the road, and we are willing to pay the price, and we choose to do what will make us better, and we get the picture in our head clearly focused in high resolution without scotoma, then we are ready to talk ourselves into taking action.

CHAPTER FOUR

MASTERING MIND CONTROL

THE SCARY PART

The first four steps to mastering mind control are primarily conceptual. The last five steps center around convincing ourselves we have the internal power to attain our goal or to live our picture. The last five steps take discipline and perseverence, a willingness not to give up.

5. Engage in self-talk: talk, picture, emotion.

Denis Waitley contributed greatly to perfecting self-talk. Self-talk takes on four dimensions: (a) first person, (b) present tense, (c) positive and (d) action-emotion oriented.

➤ First person: Start with "I." I like myself at 180 pounds. I am excited as I feel my clothes fit loose at 180 pounds.

➤ Present tense: State it as of "now." Even though I might weigh 210 pounds, I see myself at 180 and I tell myself I am 180.

➤ Positive: Put a positive spin on it and don't lead yourself to the rock in the road. I see myself at 180, not I want or need to lose 30 pounds. Stay away from negative thoughts like, I hate myself at 210 pounds.

➤ Action-emotion oriented: Generate excitement and feeling. I see myself at 180 pounds, I feel my clothes fit loose at 180 pounds, I see people admiring me at 180 pounds, I feel light and carefree at 180 pounds, I feel women lusting for my body at 180 pounds.

The idea is to use self-talk to motivate you to do what you are telling yourself to do or to be. The more emotional you can be and the more you can feel it, the more vivid the picture becomes. Self-talk enhances the development of the image or picture you are crafting.

6. Do this for 10 seconds at a time, three times a day.

Engage in self-talk once in the morning, once at noon, and once before you go to bed. You must be convincing and you must do it religiously. Rather than focus on length of time, you emphasize the number of times and intensity. The lesson of frequency and consistency has been taught through brainwashing techniques used throughout history, as revealed by prisoners of war. Accounts of individuals being held captive have been recorded throughout time, but the most noted are those reported by Viktor Frankl, Captain Gerald Coffee, and Major William Mayer. Although many lessons are learned from POWs, the single most important lesson is how much internal strength many individuals have under seemingly dire conditions and hopeless circumstances. The importance of perseverance and the will to continue living is striking and inspirational. The flip side of this internal strength is equally as fascinating and educational.

Major William E. Mayer, a psychiatrist, conducted an exhaustive study of returning prisoners of war captured in Korea by the Chinese. The psychological methods used were deceptively simple, yet powerful and effective. Major Mayer referred to this brainwashing technique as a weapon, one as powerful as a nuclear device. The fact was, up to 4,000 Americans who survived those years of captivity in 12 separate camps were guarded often by as few as one armed guard per 100 prisoners. Never, not once in the course of the entire Korean conflict, did a single American successfully, permanently escape from any established POW camp. This has never before or after happened in the history of America. No machine gun towers, no guard dogs, no electric fences, no search lights . . . Yet nobody tried to escape because they were actually imprisoned by their own minds.

When the tired, scared prisoner entered the camp, rather than being beaten, tortured, or interrogated, they were extended a hand of friendship and welcomed by an individual who spoke their language and they were asked only to keep an open mind, listen, and not to try to resist. From that point on, the prisoners went through an intense educational regime that required listening to long lectures on topics like history, civics, politics, and economics. Following the lecture, all they were required to do was to participate in discussion groups. They didn't have to agree with the teacher's point of view, they just had to participate; however, if they did agree, they were favorably recognized. The educational process was systematic, consistent, and continuous. As time went by, the prisoners were encouraged to write and give presentations supporting the teachers' viewpoints, even if they didn't believe it. It was reported by Major Mayer that many of the prisoners saw this as a joke or sham, but did, in fact, write papers and give oral presentations, taking positions against their own personal beliefs. Over time they talked themselves into acquiescing and gave up their will to try to escape. Shockingly, some gave up their will to live. Thirty-eight percent of those captured died, the highest death rate of Americans in any kind of captivity in any prison in any way since the American Revolution. They did not die because of mass execution or systematic starvation, but primarily, many just gave up. This type of death was termed "give-up-itis." These individuals would crawl into a corner, pull a blanket over their heads, and die within hours. Not starved to death. No physical disease present. They were not psychotic. They were not insane. They knew what they were doing. They made the most profound of all human surrenders. They talked themselves into giving up to the point of death.

Obviously there were many factors involved other than just talking themselves into acquiescence, such as fear, loneliness, removal of the discontents to other camps, control of the mail, etc. However, the point must be made that many of those that died and those that continued to live actually participated, believing they were lying to themselves in order to fool the enemy but, as we have learned, the subconscious cannot distinguish fact from fiction. The subconscious has no value mechanism, it just does what it is told.

As we master our own mind control, we must keep in mind we are not prisoners of war. Therefore, we must force ourselves to continuously tell ourselves, through self-talk again and again because, over time, we will, in fact, do what we tell ourselves to do. Since we are not prisoners of war, it is simple to quit. It is easy to give up because no one is making us do anything. But the minute we stop imagining and the minute we stop our self-talk, we give up controlling our mind and begin to react to the environment. The environment controls our minds rather than us controlling our own minds. Mastering mind control is not easy; it is simple, but it is **not** easy.

7. Apply attitude, knowledge, skills.

We do not want to create a false sense of hope. Although mind control is mental and predominantly attitudinal, we need to remind ourselves that in the real world, we have knowledge and skills. I can tell myself I'm 180 pounds, but if I don't know anything about nutrition, calories, exercise, fitness, then all the talk and visioning is worthless. It has been said that attitude makes up 65 percent of our success and knowledge and skills make up the other 35 percent. It doesn't make any difference what the percentages are as long as we realize knowledge and skill are necessary to attain our desired goal. Without knowledge and skill we become PMA Freaks (Positive Mental Attitude Freaks).

8. When you fail, change your goals on the run.

If you do not occasionally fail, then probably you are not pushing yourself hard enough. The ultimate challenge when using mind control is to determine our limits. However, when we do fail, we want to get back on track as soon as possible. Everyone has experienced a slump or a streak of bad luck. Why is that if we fail once, we usually fail repeatedly? One of the major reasons is because it is so hard to get back on track. Once we fail, it is hard to get the failure out of our head. We mentally see the failure clearer than we envision success; we lead ourselves to the rock in the road. The first step to getting back on track is to flush the failure out of our mind by using self-talk. Immediately after we fail, we tell ourselves, "That's not like me. That's not the Jim Payne I know." Then we follow this personal reprimand self-talk with positive self-talk, directing us toward our picture.

It is the World Series, Yankees vs. Dodgers, 1978. Ninth inning, two out, two on. The count is three-and-two. The batter is Reggie Jackson; the pitcher is a rookie, Bob Welch. Tension mounts as millions watch on T.V. Reggie Jackson, named Mr. October because he always performed under pressure, especially in October during the World Series, fouls off one, two, three balls, then suddenly strikes out. The Yankees lose, but what everyone remembers is Reggie threw a God-awful temper tantrum. He pounded the bat to the ground, raised his fists in the air, ranted, raved, cursed, yelled, stomped and, to many, made an ass of himself. Those who knew him, however, knew he was flushing that failure out of his mind and shortly thereafter he would begin to mentally prepare himself for next time.

The next time Jackson faced Bob Welch, no contest — homerun.

Let's imagine for a moment what it must be like to play with a person of Reggie Jackson's caliber. Think for a moment what must happen every time he strikes out — a swinging strike. He stomps back to the dugout, jams the bat into the rack, sits down on the bench, curses at himself, and fumes for a few seconds. If you were stupid enough to go over and try to console him by patting him on his back and saying "That is O.K. Reggie you'll get it next time," he would push you away, scowl at you and shout, "Get out of my face, don't lead me to failure." Within time, he gets composure. He focuses on the pitcher. You see the intensity in his eyes. His forearms are on his knees, thumbs pressed against his forefingers, and he is imagining ball down — bat around — ball explode; ball down — bat around — ball explode; ball down — bat around — ball explode . . . . He is mentally preparing himself for success **after** he has flushed failure out of his mind. By the time he gets up to bat again, he has successfully, mentally, hit more than 100 pitches. Reggie Jackson, Mr. October, is a master of mind control. Reggie Jackson hit five actual homeruns in one World Series, and heaven only knows how many mental ones he hit.

Twenty years ago I took Louis Tice's New Age Thinking course. As I completed the course, I realized one thing that constantly, continuously made me angry was that I couldn't keep track of my car keys. I'd lose my car keys all the time. Every time I misplaced the keys, I'd accuse someone of moving them and when I finally would find them, I'd tell myself I could never remember my keys. Through the work of Tice's program, I realized I was leading myself to failure. I pictured myself not being able to remember my keys. I'd self-talk myself into not remembering my keys. I believed I couldn't remember my keys, thus, I couldn't find my keys. Then, I realized, I'm of normal intelligence, my mind is normal, I have a decent memory, so I made up my mind to remember my keys. When I shut off the car, I would immediately remove the keys and put them on my belt and I would say to myself, "Keys on belt, keys on belt, keys on belt . . . ." The first time I misplaced my keys, when I found them, I scolded myself, "That's not like me, that's not the Jim Payne I know, I'm of normal intelligence, I can remember things." Then I grabbed the keys, thrust them on my belt, and said "keys on belt, keys on belt, keys on belt." Do you realize, prior to Tice's course, I misplaced my keys all the time and after the course, I've only misplaced the keys twice, at which time I flushed the mishap out of my mind and programmed myself for success. Twenty years later, I continue to remember where my keys are. I always have my keys on my belt when I'm not driving and I'm proud of it. It makes me feel good about myself as I confidently retrieve my keys from my belt. I like myself better. I have a better self-image of myself. I never misplace my keys, never. Now, sometimes I don't know where my car is, but I always can find my keys.

Let's say you are working on something and you continue to fail. The rule of thumb is, if you continue to fail for 7 to 10 days, you should do something different because your mind won't let you continue to tell yourself something that isn't true. Remember, you are not a prisoner of war. No one is forcing you to continue, so you will stop your self-talk. Before stopping your self-talk, change your goals on the run. Move your goal closer.

Example: "I see myself at 180 pounds, I like myself at 180 pounds, I see women lusting . . . ." But five days later I step on the scales and I weight 215 pounds–I've **gained** five pounds. Changing my goals on the run, "I see myself at 195 pounds, I like myself at 195 pounds, I see . . ." You get the idea.

9. Measure the outcome — feedback.

The last step is nothing more than a feedback or monitoring process that helps us keep on track. When possible, it is helpful if we can measure our progress objectively. This can be done in numbers or percentages. Most skill development can be measured as to accuracy, amount, length, speed, etc. Sometimes a vivid clear picture is selected that can't be measured objectively, so subjective judgment comes into play.

An example where judgment could be considered is improving one's ability to speak or improving an ability to interact with others. In these cases, it is necessary for us to get a feel for what we are doing in real life and if we think we are getting better, then we are, in fact, getting better. The beauty of using judgment is that we are the only ones we have to please. In addition to using our own judgment, sometimes we can monitor ourselves by video taping or audio taping our behavior or performance. If we are fortunate to have an objective friend that is knowledgeable as to what we are attempting to improve upon, we might find their comments helpful. The purpose of the feedback is to help the creative subconscious maneuver toward the target.

Now that we know the nine steps to mastering mind control, we can get started. Keep in mind that any time we feel awkward, uneasy or tense, this indicates we are beginning to move out of our comfort zone. These times of awkwardness, tenseness, or stressfulness help define our frame surrounding our comfort zone. These uneasy times also might indicate areas we might consider working on.

Remember, if it is to be, it is up to me.

The law of expectation is: experience shows that we seldom, if ever, exceed our expectations.

You get what you expect. What are you expecting?

CHAPTER FIVE

MASTERING MIND CONTROL FOR REAL

t was my sixth year of teaching at the University of Virginia and the course syllabus, text, and assignments were the same as the previous five years: attend class, read the text, apply visual imagery/mental rehearsal to something in your life for six weeks, and write it up in a paper of no more than 10 pages in length using the American Psychological Association format.

Two weeks into the course, Mary Jane Ellis appeared at my office, a blonde, squeaky clean, preppie-looking young lady. After sitting down, she flippantly began to explain it was not working, referring to the visual imagery/mental rehearsal assignment.

She was trying to apply it to making herself jog every morning after she got up. She explained, "Before I go to bed I engage in self-talk as you explained in class — first person, present tense, positive and action-emotion oriented. I like myself as I jog, I see myself jogging, I feel my body getting hot as I jog... You know, the stuff you said in class. I do the same thing when I wake up, but I just roll over and go back to sleep."

I made a feeble attempt to tell her she had to put a little effort into it, that the self-talk wasn't something magic. It wouldn't make you physically jump out of bed, but I saw she wasn't paying a lot of attention, so I quickly concluded, "Just continue for the total of six weeks, write it up. Your grade is not dependent on positive results. I'm mainly interested that you just try it." Somewhat nonresponsive, she got up from the chair and left.

Three weeks later, she came down in front of the lecture hall and said to me, "I've got it working." To be honest, there were more than 300 students in the class and I just vaguely remembered her, but I didn't have a clue what she was talking about.

At the end of the semester, I started reading this stack of papers, some of which were interesting and some not so interesting, and all of a sudden I came to this paper that was three times the length of the other papers. It was Mary Jane's. In the paper she explained what she was attempting to do, described the procedure, mentioned coming to my office and returning to her apartment and continuing the procedure for a few days without any success. Then she began to explain in emotional terms her disgust with herself and that she was spoiled, and her anger at herself for being so lazy that she just wouldn't get up in the morning and jog. She used terms like slob, lazy ass, degenerate, bitch, and other less complimentary names. She went on to explain she was born into a wealthy family and she would never have to work and she wondered why she was attending school — it was a waste of time for her and everyone else. Suddenly, the paper shifted direction and she began to explain as a "poor little rich kid" she had value and was better than just being a slob. She explained she realized why the self-talk wasn't working, in her own words: "Suddenly I realized the reason the self-talk wasn't working was because it wasn't real for me. I couldn't see it, I couldn't feel it — they were just words. I thought it was a joke."

As I continued to read this self-confession, this self-analysis, she began to explain how she made the self-talk become meaningful. One afternoon she forced herself to jog and, as she jogged, she recorded her heavy breathing in a portable tape recorder. That night, as she went to sleep, she would begin her self-talk while listening to herself breathe using the recording as background noise. After completing the self-talk, she would continue to listen to herself huff and puff on the tape until she fell asleep. The tape recorder would automatically shut off at the conclusion of the tape. She claimed that in the morning, when her alarm went off, she would spring from her bed, put on her jogging outfit and, as she engaged in self-talk, she would proceed to go out and jog before breakfast. This continued every morning until the paper was due.

After completing the paper, I didn't know whether to believe it or not and wondered if she was pulling my leg. Realizing I didn't have time to validate the authenticity of every paper, I graded it, taking points off for not following the requirement of limiting it to ten pages.

Much to my surprise, Mary Jane Ellis came to my office after the course was completed to thank me for teaching her about herself. This time I remembered her and her paper and if she was pulling my leg, she was very good at it. I thanked her for her kind comments and for taking the course and, for some reason, mentioned if she had time, I'd like to listen to the tape she used for background noise. Later that afternoon she returned with the tape and tape recorder. She sat down and the two of us listened to the tape. Sure enough, it was nothing more than her breathing. No music, no narration, just breathing and, toward the end, it was almost hyper ventilating. Admittedly, I was surprised at the tape and fascinated at the procedure for making the self-talk become more meaningful.

A year later Mary Jane wrote me a letter indicating she was still jogging every morning. We became pen pals and unfortunately her father passed away unexpectedly and she took over the family business in Atlanta. Ten years later she continues to jog every morning, even in inclement weather. She attributed her discipline, pride, and perseverence applied to jogging carried into successfully running the company. For Mary Jane, visual imagery/mental rehearsal continued over time and carried over to other parts of her life. This may be why some refer to this self-motivation field as the field of personal development.

Another case I was involved with dealt with Melvin Seamore. Melvin was five foot ten inches, weighed 140 pounds, and wanted to increase his upper body strength. Simply put, he wanted to get girls. Melvin chose working out in the weight room for his project.

Melvin Seamore was a rather shy, reserved young man. He called for an appointment and arrived at the exact appointed time. He explained his frustration, that he was intimidated by the idea of going to the weight room to work out. He would engage in self-talk, go to the weight room, but would only half-heartedly work out, because, as he put it, everyone would look at him out of the corner of their eyes as if to say, What is this guy doing in here?

I explained, since he was at least going to the weight room, maybe he could alter his self-talk to include working more vigorously and for longer stretches of time. He indicated he had tried, but felt intimidated. He went on to explain he didn't understand why the people that were in the weight room were there. They really didn't need to be there. They all looked great. He was the only one who could be identified as a little skinny punk.

Rather than handing his paper in like the rest of the students, he brought his by personally. He wanted to thank me in person and explain how he gained ten pounds and increased his upper body strength just within a semester's time.

According to Melvin, to increase his motivation, he had his roommate take Polaroid pictures of him lifting weights. One good front view and one good side view. Next, he used the same sweat socks each day in the weight room, but never washed them. At night, before going to sleep, he would engage in self-talk as he laid in bed. While talking to himself, he would look at the two pictures — front and side view — imagining himself bigger, stronger, and more handsome. After completing the self-talk, he would lay the pictures down on the night stand next to the bed and promptly pick up the sweat socks and smell them before dropping off to sleep. He said the stench of the socks made his vision of lifting weights in the weight room more vivid and real. Melvin emphatically proclaimed this procedure inspired him to lift weights longer and with greater intensity.

What Mary Jane and Melvin taught me was for individuals that may have difficulty using the self-talk to create their picture and make it more vivid and real, when they involved other senses, like smelling, hearing, touching, and seeing, it helps. Later, I found as individuals used their senses to magnify their vision of themselves, physiological changes took place that could be objectively measured. As a person sees, smells, hears or touches while engaging in self-talk, their pulse rate may actually increase or decrease and their temperature rise or fall. If a person can actually get a physiological change to occur in their body by just thinking about it, then it doesn't take too much of an imagination to realize this self-talk stuff is for real and not just hocus-pocus or pop psychology. My most striking case was Betty.

Betty explained to me she was under psychiatric care for severe depression and she had tried to commit suicide twice; once by taking an over dose of sleeping pills and then again by cutting her wrists with a razor blade. The depression was triggered when her boyfriend jilted her. She was very much in love with him and continued to be infatuated with him. I couldn't understand her feelings for him, because she told me that he physically abused her and psychologically mistreated her. Still, she loved him. Every time she thought about losing him, she would become depressed. She targeted the reduction of her depression for her class project. Her concern was, since she had started her self-talk to flush Sylvester out of her mind, the number of depression episodes and the severity of her depression had increased. I explained that since she was receiving professional help and since this involved her physical safety and well-being, she should choose another topic for her paper. She listened, nodded, and quietly left the office.

A week later she came to my office and explained she was still trying to use self-talk to reduce her depression and it was getting a little better. She said she realized her original self-talk of flushing Sylvester out of her mind was really a violation of step one, get a picture of what you want — not what you don't want. As she tried to talk herself into ridding her mind of Sylvester, she was actually leading herself to the rock in the road. Now she was focusing on seeing herself happy, contented, and doing purposeful things.

During the last week of the semester Betty burst into my office unannounced. She joyfully explained that for the past two weeks she was able to sleep without interruption and she had experienced no deep depression. She explained, "Two weeks ago I was tossing and turning in bed and I got so depressed I decided to kill myself. I went to the bathroom, took out a razor blade, and just as I was about to slit my wrists, I looked up into the mirror to see a crying, frantic, pathetic young woman at her wit's end, and I realized it was me. Suddenly, I thought, neither Sylvester, nor any man, is worth taking my life for."

She continued, "I don't know what made me do it, but I dropped the razor blade into the trash basket, washed my face off with a cold, damp wash cloth, walked to my desk, sat down, took out a piece of paper, and wrote at the top of the paper 'BETTY'S PERSONAL MENU.' Then I began to list the things that were dear to me, things that made life worth living. The most important thing to me was my mom and dad. They had stuck by my side through thick and thin and never wavered. I wrote #1. MOM & DAD. Then I pictured them smiling at me and looking at me with their caring, loving eyes. Oh, they are so important to me. Next, I thought of my sister. She is so supportive, helpful, and encouraging. I wrote #2. SISTER. We are truly buddies. Next, I thought of my job. I have a good job and my boss is concerned about me and tolerant and patient. I wrote #3. JOB. Everyone at work likes me and cares about me. Finally, I think what else is worth living for, what turns me on, what excites me? Suddenly, I write #4. PEANUT CLUSTER. I laughed as I wrote peanut cluster, but I love the taste of chocolate and peanuts. I imagine the taste and I feel the crunch as I bite down into a peanut cluster. I'm in heaven. Suddenly, I got up from the desk and went to the refrigerator and got me three peanut clusters. I lay down in bed and, as I devoured the peanut clusters, I thought of all the good times I've had with my family and friends. Contented, I fell asleep and never stirred until the alarm went off. I got up, looked at my personal menu, engaged in some positive self-talk, had breakfast and, while driving to work, ate three more peanut clusters.

"During work, at about ten, I started to go into a little depression. I immediately went to the bathroom, took out of my purse my personal menu, engaged in self-talk, and, before gong back out on the floor, I secured a peanut cluster from a baggie filled with peanut clusters I had placed in my purse. I ate it ever so slowly. I was at peace with myself and I reveled in the chocolate.

"Throughout the week, I continued this ritual and, suddenly, I realized I didn't need to actually eat the peanut cluster. I could just think about eating it. Within days I realized I didn't need to read my actual personal menu, it was enough just to think about mom, dad, sister, job, peanut cluster. For two weeks I controlled my own mind."

As you read about Betty, you realize the personal menu and the stupid peanut cluster thing really worked. Betty kept in contact with me and occasionally we still communicate with one another. She is a happy, well-balanced, mother and has a very fine husband who, by the way, is not Sylvester. She no longer needs psychotherapy and she teaches visual imagery and mental rehearsal, as a Girl Scout mother to her Girl Scout troop.

I am sitting in the Red Roof Inn. Watched television for forty-five minutes and have no idea of what I've watched because all I could see or think about was that policeman. Tight shirt, badge, gun, boots, and hat. I hate policemen. Suddenly, I go to the desk, take out some Red Roof Inn stationary, and I write at the top: JAMES S. PAYNE PERSONAL MENU. #1. MOM & DAD. They are so wonderful, next to Godliness. #2. MY FAMILY. KIM, JANET. What would I do without them? They are what I live for. #3. JOB. What a job, I'm actually paid to teach and serve. Can you believe they actually pay me to do the things I love to do? I pause, think, reflect, and write: #4. REESE'S PEANUT BUTTER CUP. Wow, what a heavenly taste. It makes my mouth water now, even as I write it down to share it with you.

Now, as you read the true stories of Betty and me and the policeman, you realize, when you start to let something get you down you can immediately change the course of your true thoughts and feelings by consciously forcing yourself to focus on the positives in your life. The personal menu trick has worked for me time and time again. And, like Betty, I don't need to write it out I can just think about it. This is the trick you can use to control your own dreams if you so choose.

The next time you wake up from a bad dream, take a moment to collect some positive thoughts and images. Begin some simple self-talk and allow yourself to fall back to sleep as you pleasantly imagine those things in your life that are of high value. You will feel a calmness and tranquility fall over you. You will become enveloped in a euphoric state. You will actually float into a state of unconsciousness and you will begin to dream pleasant, positive dreams in living color.

After you do this a couple of times, you may decide to control all your dreams and, if you do, you will realize that with very little practice and a lot of discipline, you will become a skilled master of controlling your dreams. At this point, you truly have mastered mind control.

My wife of 38 years passed away less than a year ago. On occasion, I catch myself dreaming about her. Whether the dream is positive or negative, invariably, when I wake up, I begin to go through slight depression. Just as I start to get those sad, empty, depressing feelings, I abruptly free

myself to visually picture good, joyous times with my daughters (I sometimes look at photos I have of them displayed in the bedroom), vividly
imagine a wonderful time I had with my granddaughter (again, I may
simultaneously look at a picture of her), and finally revel in the pleasure
of mentally touching, smelling, and tasting a Reese's Peanut Butter Cup.
These quick three mental photo snapshots take less than two minutes
and erases or flushes out the depressive thoughts and ideas triggered by
the dream. If it is early morning, I roll over, begin to envision something
I'm going to do in the future that is very pleasurable, like visit my daughters, take my granddaughter to a show, play golf with my friends, or possibly dine at a fine restaurant, and then I go back to sleep. If it is late
morning and too late to go back to sleep, I get up, shower, dress, and eat
breakfast. While showering, I envision something positive I'm going to do
in the near future. I strongly advise that if you have not already used this
technique, try it. It works for me each and every time. It takes mental
effort and discipline. It is simple but not easy, and with very little practice, it can be mastered quickly.

PART II:
MENTAL STAIRCASE
(MOTIVATION OF OTHERS)

CHAPTER SIX

Not All Minds Are the Same

learn a lot on airplanes. On a return flight from a conference about motivation, a young man seated next to me shared a lesson more useful than many lessons learned at the conference. He explained:

"I remember back when I was on the high school football team. I was the assistant water boy. We had a very strong team and I was too small to play, but I wanted to be a part of the team anyway.

We were into our third game and playing this team that was supposed to be real easy. Well, at half-time the score was 21-0, their favor. We were supposed to be running all over them, but we weren't. Everybody crept into the locker room at the half and sheepishly sat down. We sat on the benches just looking down and, oh goodness, we didn't want Coach to come in. We didn't know what was going to happen, but we knew it wasn't going to be good.

You could hear a pin drop in that locker room. Coach didn't say anything, just went over and picked up a stool and hurled that rascal the full length of the locker room. It crashed into the wall and broke into a hundred pieces. We looked up and he started into one of the most motivational talks I've ever heard. We knocked down the door getting out of the locker room and back to the game.

To tell the truth, I don't remember whether we won or lost, but I can tell you, that team had all the water they could possibly drink in the second half."

Later, I discovered that this was a popular story attributed to Willie Gayle, a famous lecturer on motivation. Regardless of where the story originated, it's a good illustration of how motivation reaches every level in an organization. But motivating is a two-edged sword.

A number of years ago, another football team discovered that many of the more aggressive players were drinking too much water and were getting sluggish during practice. The result was sloppy performance. Management hired a nutritionist whose solution was to allocate water based on a complicated formula using temperature, humidity, activity, and player body weight.

At first, they tried dispensing the water in soufflé cups, about the size of a jigger. During time-outs, a trainer was to run onto the field carrying a cafeteria tray with the correct number of little cups. You can imagine presenting soufflé cups full of water to mean, tough, hyped-up, sweaty, and thirsty interior linemen. This was psychologically insulting. The well-intended plan resulted in unhappy players and soufflé cups knocked all over the place. The anger turned against management instead of against rival teams. Motivation can be destructive as well as constructive — the two-edged sword.

From this fiasco came the squirt bottle. Players could go to the sidelines and fill up; or, better yet, the trainer could run onto the field and squirt water into their mouths. Squirt, squirt, squirt — it was like filling their tanks. Squirt, squirt, they loved it, and it was still relatively simple to regulate the intake of water. The team turned water intake back into a positive motivator. Many of the players viewed themselves as machines — big, powerful machines — that had to be tanked up to run.

With the advent of Gatorade and other electrolyte-balancing fluids, water-sluggishness is less of a problem. Yet, sideline liquids still teach us about motivation. Not all players handle their Gatorade the same way — people are different.

Watch a big offensive lineman walk up to the cooler. He'll grab a cup, jam it under the spigot, turn it on, then leave it on! Some offensive linemen like to watch stuff pour all over the ground, or possibly on their shoes. After a while, they'll stop the flow, gulp their drink, then smash the cup and head back to the game.

Quarterbacks are different. They'll fill a cup half-full, study the game while it breathes, then sip slowly. They're also less likely to be doing the post-game cooler-dump on the coach. Does that mean quarterbacks are nicer than linemen? Or that linemen aren't as nice to their mothers? No, but it's more evidence that people are different, and that there's more to those differences than pure randomness.

Each of us carries a mental blueprint or picture of who we are. All of our actions, feelings, behaviors — even our abilities — are consistent with our picture of who we believe we are. In short, we act like the sort of person we perceive ourselves to be. One neat motivational trick is to amplify compatible actions and things that reinforce our picture — squirt bottles for those that see themselves as powerful machines, light paper cups for those that see themselves as football surgeons. This is brain-to-brain motivation.

There are no such things as unmotivated persons, as long as they're breathing. It is easy for people to find motivation to do the things they enjoy. Brain-to-brain motivation helps people do things they don't ordinarily enjoy doing. It is easy to get someone to do something they like or want to do. Getting someone to do something they don't like or don't want to do is a different story.

Many people believe that money motivates every adult. If you can get the ante high enough, you can get anyone to do anything. Research and experience don't bear this out. Loyalty, prestige, friendship, purpose, love, fear, praise, and a host of other things work, too.

The old stereotypes imply that all children can be motivated by candy. It wasn't true in the "good old days," and it's certainly not the case in this age of nutritional awareness. Either literally or symbolically, there is no great candy bar in the sky, no cosmic M&M that gets a positive response from everyone. People are different.

People differ in how they view things and in what they believe. Consider the possible ways to see . . .

- law and order
- marriage and family
- religion
- quality of life
- morality

People also differ in how they act. Look at the cars we drive (or want to drive). Some for status, some for safety, others for inexpensive transportation, and some for comfort. Look at the clothes people wear (or would like to wear). Some to fit in, some to stand out, and others for pure function. Look at how people live. Some to maintain order, others to break free; some to join together, others to stand alone.

Yet all these different people often must work together and find ways to achieve common goals. To assist various individuals in accomplishing and completing often distasteful tasks while simultaneously enjoying what they are doing, or at least minimizing the dissatisfaction, we turn to **PeopleWise® Motivation.**

Oftentimes, we expect others to react and respond and come to the same conclusions as we do from a given set of facts or circumstances. We must constantly keep reminding ourselves that no one reacts to things as they are, but only as they believe them, or see them, or imagine them to be. As we master the art of motivating brain-to-brain, we get on the same wavelength.

PeopleWise® Motivation recognizes that people are different — they should not, cannot, and must not be treated identically. It's unfair to treat all people just alike, because that denies them the right to their unique strengths and competencies. An effective motivation system must first account for differences before it attempts to coordinate diversity.

I once worked with vacuum cleaner salespeople who prospected customers through several "cold canvas" phone calls. There aren't many salespeople — vacuum cleaner, insurance, real estate, or automobile — who really enjoy making cold calls. Some can be motivated to find this distasteful task more acceptable through extensive training in telephone skills and desensitization. Others may respond when incentives are applied, such as paying a bonus for every 10 completed phone calls.

However, a particular salesperson in the group wasn't motivated by training, money, threat, or harassment. This gal just wouldn't use the phone. She claimed she wanted to, wasn't afraid to, and knew how important it was. But she still didn't make her quota of calls.

After a couple of interviews, I discovered she was quite opinionated and rather religious. She enjoyed listening to hymns and liked marching music. She was also committed to doing her job and was willing to experiment with personal motivation.

First, we recorded several of her favorite hymns and marches on a cassette. Next, she disciplined herself to sit at the phone and make five quick calls first thing every morning. After the calls, she'd turn on the tape player and march around the desk three times as *Onward Christian Soldiers* rang out across the room. Another song and another parade and she'd do five more. Soon she was making more calls than any other salesperson, was more enthusiastic while she made her calls, and she became the best producer in the company. In short, she became motivated to do something she didn't like or want to do and, once motivated, she learned to like it a little.

A similar approach worked for a track star. He didn't enjoy weight training, but found that by listening to the theme from *Rocky*, just prior and sometimes during his exercise program, he not only tolerated the lifting but began to look forward to it. He found he was able to stay with the task longer and tolerate doing a distasteful task.

Through brain-to-brain motivation, the salesperson developed a habit of making cold calls. Through brain-to-brain motivation, the track star developed the habit of exercise through weight training. Habits help us clarify our pictures. It is impossible to develop a habit outside our picture. To make a distasteful action become a habit, we must either move the habit into the picture or move the picture to the habit. The word "habit" originally meant garment or clothing. This gives us an insight into the true meaning of habit. Our habits are literally garments worn by us. They fit and they, over time, become a part of us. When the habit is no longer a part of us we quit doing the task. Brain-to-Brain Motivation puts the habit in the picture or moves the picture to the habit.

The point is, people see things differently. They view the world through different lenses. The problem is, if people are so different and unique, it seems impossible to know what should and shouldn't be done. Fortunately, while it's true that people are unique, most normal people behave rationally and most interactions are not chaotic when we understand the pattern of thought processes behind the actions. **PeopleWise®** **Motivation** helps us understand those thinking systems and decision structures. Once you recognize how people think and what really matters, you realize there is an internal logic behind what they do. You may not agree or like it, but you can begin to understand. After you understand it, you become better at motivating them brain-to-brain.

CHAPTER SEVEN

Minds Expand Along Predictable Staircase Steps

During a biology course I took at Dodge City Jr. College, in the 1950s, my instructor, Professor Sites, described three different theories to explain the same event. How could this be? Three different explanations of a singular outcome. Surely one was right and the other two erroneous.

When challenged, Dr. Sites stated that theories are nothing more than ways of thinking about a thing. They are frameworks that support and structure ideas. In the words of Professor Sites,

> Theories are not truths — say not "it is the truth," but say, "so it seems to me to be, as I now see the thing I think I see."

Semanticist Alfred Korzybski made the same point by saying the map is not the territory. This book is a map to the things we think we see and an atlas of how we see them. It doesn't pretend to offer the truth; but it will give you a revolutionary way to get at the truth. Once you've got this framework and master a few basic principles, you will be able (a) to understand the differences in people's thinking and then (b) to shop among alternative motivation tools for the ones which will fit the people and situation best.

Theories do three things:

1. They make sense out of apparent chaos;
2. They allow us to predict things beyond chance; and
3. They lead us to key variables which, if altered, result in changed outcomes.

Good behavioral theories help us make things happen rather than passively letting things happen to us. In this case, we're after better, more effective motivation. It's easy enough to observe what people do. Understanding their actions is tougher. Theories help us fill in the reasons **why** and then lead us to **what to do.**

If productivity drops, we want to know why: "His work has deteriorated because the supervisor's constant put-downs are ego-deflating" or, "her quality's down because she doesn't feel like there's much opportunity for a woman to advance in that department." As a theory begins to clarify what's going on, it begins to predict: "He'll get mad and really pull back if it goes on much longer" or, "We'll lose her unless she sees more ways to make things happen." A useful theory then suggests ways to make things happen: "We can reassign that supervisor to a group that's more compatible with his rough-and-tumble style" or, "Let's involve her in this company-wide project to demonstrate some options."

PeopleWise® Motivation gives you a way to (a) make some sense out of all the crazy things that happen with, to, and about people; (b) predict how certain people are likely to react to given conditions; and (c) provide options to consider when deciding what to do.

It is important to have a psychological match between people's expectations and the motivation approaches used with them. It happens in the workplace and in the home. Different people think about the same thing in different ways. One person wants just to get the job done while the other wants to think on it, meditate about it, and consider options. One spouse wants to eat; the other wants to dine. One wants to buy; the other wants to shop. One wants sex; the other wants romance. In a way, we have the same wants and needs, but our thinking is out of sync. The same thing happens between unions and management or politicians and their constituencies.

There are a number of very popular and familiar theories which offer explanations of this match/mismatch phenomenon. For instance, Blake and Mouton's classic Managerial Grid, "McGregor's Theory X & Y," "Myers-Briggs Personality Types," "Block's Empowered Manager," "Deming's work on quality and continuous improvement," and even Tom Peters' various manifestations of excellence, offer explanations of what puts things in and out of sync.

All of the above examples have merit, but a difficulty with these approaches is that they rely on snapshots instead of flows. That's why so much of management (and education, and parenting, and rehabilitation, and coaching) leaves a lot to be desired. Individuals are neither lazy nor exuberant, responsible nor irresponsible, enamored of work nor reluctant to work. They are all of these things, constantly changing, always in process.

The late Dr. Clare W. Graves, professor, Union College at Schenectady, New York, believed that humankind is psychologically evolving. Sometimes we like work and sometimes we don't; some of us are responsible and others aren't; and furthermore, most individuals change as time goes by. But change is not random, magical, or unfathomable. Graves found an elegant pattern beneath the seeming chaos of human existence. His 30 years of research disclosed a predictable psychological hierarchy, a series of layers through which we may pass. When individual needs are appropriately met, wherever they happen to lie in the stack, people will not only tend to be productive but will even enjoy working, learning, and living. They can be motivated.

The theory behind **PeopleWise® Motivation** is based on Graves' pioneering research. This is not a theory book and we won't go into it at great depth, but we believe one should be familiar with some of the background. In the early 1950s, Clare Graves began asking the question, "What makes a mature adult personality?" There were many answers and theories. He wasn't satisfied with them, though. Most were based on typologies for people, categories, and little boxes. Graves wasn't convinced that people existed so simply as fixed types. He'd seen too many people change over time. And he couldn't draw sharp lines between them; the idea of X number of pure types, whatever the magic number, just didn't seem to make sense.

Furthermore, the models were descriptive, not predictive. Graves wanted to understand not only where people were in their thinking, but where they were likely to go next — movies, not snapshots. He wanted to explore the flow of human development, not just to lump people into a few groups. His friend and colleague, Abraham Maslow, had built a model based around a Hierarchy of Needs. These needs ranged from very basic subsistence through a state called self-actualization. The model was visualized as a pyramid people climbed as they developed from physiological needs to security, to safety, to love, to esteem, to self-actualization.

Graves saw a glitch in Maslow's work. To really understand what people do, and why they do it, you have to factor in how they see the world and what the world they're in is like. "Self-actualization" has to be taken in context. "Mature" thinking for one group or situation is quite inappropriate for another. Moreover, you have to factor in their natural brain equipment and intelligences. Though all normal human brains have great potential, they aren't the same. Furthermore, we don't seem to share capacities in equal measure. Talents, instincts, gifts, and "naturals" at this or that distinguish people and must be taken into account in any good motivation system.

For a quarter century, he quietly conducted experiments, gathered data, and refined his ideas. He worked in the business community and the classroom. Sometimes, even his colleagues at Union College were unknowing subjects. He was able to follow some of his subjects for years — from college sophomore to corporate executive, parent, nurse, or military officer — and to observe how and why and when they changed.

Although his approach was unique, Clare Graves was not alone in the quest to understand what motivates people. However, he stands apart because his work is the most comprehensive; all the other models can fit within his framework, but no other is powerful enough to encompass all of Graves. Part of that lies in the elegance of his longitudinal research design. Study the same people long enough across a variety of situations and you can discover a lot. Part also lies in his own character. Graves always claimed to be one of those folks with an "odd" brain, different somehow, as it combines information into new patterns. While others counted parts, he saw wholes. Graves' Emergent-Cyclical Levels of Psychological Development, coupled with the discipline of personal development, referred to as visual imagery and mental rehearsal, form the foundation of **PeopleWise® Motivation: The Art of Motivating Brain-to-Brain.**

PeopleWise® Motivation looks at living as an open-ended process, like a long staircase with an infinite number of steps with identifiable landings. The climb is hierarchical, emerging from less comprehensive thinking to more elaborate thinking through a predictable sequence. People can stop in a zone of comfort (landing) or continue the climb throughout their lives. In general, our species is moving farther upstairs as more expansive ways of thinking emerge.

The staircase tends to spiral between Individualist/Elitist ways of thinking and Communal/Collective views. These switches between me-orientation and we-focus play central roles in child development, cultural evolution, management, and motivation. Life can be different, depending on whether one's focus is on the "me" or the "we." You can see how important this is for management and social engineers. Some of the greatest debates of the age — abortion, ethnic education, gun control, productivity, and health care — are between the me and we factions, people operating from different levels on the staircase.

One of the simplest but most useful conclusions is that people will tell you how they want to be handled, treated, or managed. Sometimes you can get the information if you just come right out and ask; otherwise, you might have to make the determination more indirectly through interviews or surveys; but the information's there if we know how to get it.

Graves once said, "Damn it all, a person has a right to be." It's central to this point of view that there are many good, legitimate, contributing ways of being within the wide spectrum of humankind. There is no "best" way to think, nor an end-state of development. Thus, it is not our job to try to change who people are. Goodness knows, we have no business playing God anyway. What we can do is open opportunities for people to change and facilitate the process; but you can't "push the river." That's where **PeopleWise® Motivation** comes in.

The majority of people think they're somewhat special and want to be recognized as such. Although they're all selfish and egocentric at times, most of them recognize that no organization or business is structured around their every desire. They know there is some give and take in every situation. The challenge for most organizations is finding ways to integrate the meeting of individuals' needs with objectives of the collective organization.

PeopleWise® Motivation lays out specific strategies which allow us to stress both production and personal growth and development. At each step along the developmental staircase is a unique pattern of actions, feelings, ethics, and motivations. Each place has an optimal motivational system. The catch is, we stand on several steps at once. As we climb, we don't forget where we've been. Just as when we paint a porch, we add new layers of complexity on the surface, but the base-coats are still there. We carry our history with us. With the move to each new step we re-evaluate what life's all about, what our role in it is, and what constitutes a good job, marriage, etc.

There are things which set each human apart, like fingerprints and DNA profiles. However, there are also things that pull us together, common themes we share to varying degrees. We tend to bunch up at the landings. As we encounter problems on the job, at home, or in the community, we tend to deal with them from the position we're experiencing at that period in our lives. What we know sets us apart; how we think draws us together.

There's no law that says everybody has to keep climbing the stairs. We move on to another step when we get new information that forces us to question our assumptions about life and who we are. Life is a constant process of problems and solutions. Each step on the staircase, and ultimately each landing, has its own set of problems and solutions, including those that came before and those which add something new, a "yes, all that, but this too ...." statement. People don't start climbing until they've taken care of the problems where they are. Sometimes, they even have to step down when things they once resolved crop up again.

The landings are also characterized by unique coping equipment. These are the means we can access for dealing with the problems. The more complex the problems, the more complex the equipment required to deal with them. If problems outstrip equipment, we're in trouble because our tools are inadequate. If, by chance, equipment outpaces problems, you find people with bored brains — under-employed, under-achieving, and wasted. Stability at each landing means there's a matched set of problems and equipment.

One more word about equipment. **PeopleWise® Motivation** presumes that normal human brains have a great deal of potential to utilize more complex ways of thinking. Minds don't develop unless more complex problems become important and stimulate the thinking. Minds don't develop if undernourished, either. It's absolutely essential to feed young brains for them to develop to normal potential, and to feed adult brains to maintain their full capacity.

Don't get the idea that landings mean repertoires of behavior — for instance, if a person drives a Volvo, stops for red lights at 4 p.m., is an autocratic manager, or wears only brown suits. **PeopleWise® Motivation** doesn't work like that. These landings are decision-making structures — ways of thinking about things — within the person or organization. They're how we make choices, not the choices themselves.

A description for a landing is more like this:

> Thinks in true-false, right-wrong terms. Needs structure and a clear-cut chain-of-command. Learns best from respected higher authority. Motivated by fear of punishment and accepts deferred rewards. Has a linear, sequential, particularized concept of time.

This description tells us how the person thinks, but not what the person believes. It indicates why a person might act, but doesn't categorize what the person can do. Once understood, you'll see that it places the thinking within the hierarchy (on the developmental staircase) and shows what comes before (the person's back-up style or previous steps and landings) as well as what the next developmental step will be if/when movement occurs. You don't suddenly get a whole new person, but a person who's activated something new within the self.

That still sounds a little vague, but consider the awesome implications. Once you begin to understand the 'hows' and 'whys', the 'whats' become predictable. The landings tell us what kind of motivation system, what sort of organizational structure, and what educational method will be most appropriate. Each time we go through a different psychological step leading to a landing, we develop a set of different ideas about how we want to be treated, taught, managed, motivated, and even loved.

To conclude, we find humankind to be complex, changing, nonstatic, and growing. Fortunately, this maturing process develops through a series of understandable progressive steps. Once fully grasped, this process allows us not only to understand all those crazy people we see and read about that don't think or act like we do, it also lets us understand ourselves better in relation to those crazy people.

After years of studying, researching, experimenting, and applying **PeopleWise® Motivation**, we have reached a scary conclusion:

If I know you (know you psychologically) better than you know me, I can influence you.

This means, if we choose to, we can persuade others to buy something they don't need or want, get them to vote for the person we think everyone should vote for, alter their taste in food, clothes, or cars, etc.

What's even more scary is:

If I know you (psychologically know you) better than you know yourself, I can control you.

Frankly, that makes me uncomfortable. I do not want to believe anyone can control another person's life. But, after studying brain-washing techniques, terrorist tactics, and cult movements, I am saddened to report that the evidence is overwhelming; under extreme conditions, many people will psychologically break down, become weak, and allow themselves to be controlled.

Disturbing as it seems, people who don't know themselves, people who don't have a purpose in life, people who are grossly unsure of themselves can be controlled and, for the most part, are controlled regardless of environmental conditions, extreme or not.

CHAPTER EIGHT

BABY STEPS ONE AND TWO

The first step in learning the **PeopleWise®** **Motivation** system is to become acquainted with the staircase and the key landings, Levels. With the Levels clearly in mind, we can motivate people as they actually are, not as we might wish them to be or, worse yet, as mirror reflections of ourselves. In **PeopleWise®** **Motivation**, we alter the Golden Rule. We try to do unto others as they wish to be done unto.

Remember that we're not going to talk about types of people, but ways of thinking within people. There are no types of people. It's nonsense to talk about all Anglo-Saxons, or all Native-Americans, or all African-Americans, or all Chinese-Americans, as if these groups were somehow homogeneous. Instead, we'll talk about those people whose thinking is centered at a particular Level regarding a particular issue at a particular time. Within each horizontal classification scheme — race, sex, age, religion, etc. — is a vertical range of Levels. Until we begin looking at these vertical dimensions, we're still stereotyping, generalizing, and wasting time.

Let's repeat: Levels cut through ethnic groups. That's a very powerful concept because it lets us get away from discriminatory ideas and see people in a whole new light.

By understanding Levels, we can help people learn new content and expand their horizons toward new, more complex ways of thinking about that content. In other words, we can help people develop to their fullest, given who they are, and open avenues for them to grow, given who they might become. **PeopleWise®** **Motivation** is like language lessons. We learn how to speak in terms that matter to other people, helping them to find the motivators that work for them so they can learn the most with the least energy wasted. Not everyone learns the same things in the same way. **PeopleWise®** **Motivation** lets us plan education so more can be gained with less effort.

However, there's always a catch. People have different equipment. Their experiences are different and their brains are different. That means, frankly, that we all don't have equivalent access to the same ways of thinking about all things. Each person's profile is unique. This profile is not a function of age, or sex, or race, or nationality. Instead, that particular blend of DNA and life experience that makes us "us" also sets up a range of Levels or options.

Even though the normal human brain has remarkable untapped potential, everybody won't become an Einstein, or Mother Teresa, or, fortunately, Billy the Kid. There simply are no guarantees — life is full of surprises — but there are probabilities. **PeopleWise® Motivation** helps us understand these probabilities in order to make the most of who we are and what we've got. Often, we even surprise ourselves.

So let's look at the Levels found in **PeopleWise® Motivation.** You'll probably find these aspects of yourself in several of them. Most people operate with a mixture of at least two levels, and some of us even more. However, most people have a preference of how they want to be handled, how to learn, or how to think. It is also possible to step back to earlier Levels when the conditions warrant, as we sometimes do when under stress, when angry, when scared, or when we get sick.

It is not unusual for a professional athlete who is competitive, motivated to win, and who thinks strategically, to hit a slump. During the slump, anxiety goes up and the individual becomes a methodical thinker and goes back to basics and sometimes becomes superstitious.

It is not unusual for an independent person that is an adventuresome risk-taker to get ill and desire mothering.

It is not unusual for an affectionate, feeling-oriented person who experiences a threat to a loved one to become aggressive and combative.

PeopleWise® Motivation helps us understand changes in behavior by understanding changes in the thinking process. By understanding the thinking processes, mastering **PeopleWise® Motivation** becomes a reality.

To begin with, Graves found, prior to his death, eight major Levels in his research. We say "major" because, to extend the staircase metaphor, these are only the landings at the floors of human development. There are many steps in between which have their own characteristics. In other words, we're talking about an unbroken continuum which people steadily move along, not a series of types they hop between.

We'll deal with the first two rather briefly, though they represent a large part of the Earth's population. In fact, everybody reading this book has been through them. Since you're reading this book, it also means you've moved beyond them. Each of us goes through each landing until we decide to quit climbing the stairs. The first two landings are not a major part of the workplace environment, so we'll leave in-depth discussions for the more common landings/Levels. Levels 3 and above will get detailed coverage, because we can easily identify and relate with these upper Levels.

Level 1: Reactive

Level 1 is, as its number implies, the beginning. At this most basic form of human existence, thinking centers on basic physiological needs like satisfying hunger and thirst, sexual urges, and staying warm. The person really doesn't differentiate self from others. That is, the idea of "I" as a free-standing individual is not part of consciousness. There is certainly awareness of outside events and influences, but cause-and-effect links are hard to come by.

Practically all the person's energy is consumed in meeting survival needs. The biological drives and urges — eat, sleep, have sex, eliminate — are central to existence. If the person is functioning predominately at Level 1, the Level 1 brain equipment is operating in response to Level 1 conditions. That will be because —

1. Level 1 problems are all that there is in the milieu and the person is functioning appropriately (individuals isolated in the remote areas);
2. The person has not yet developed awareness of more complex problems, although they are present (infancy) or has lost contact with them (senile, elderly, mentally ill);
3. The person has limited equipment (severe retardation) or equipment that has been damaged (severe abuse, illness, accident) which may or may not be repairable.

You really don't "motivate" people at Level 1. You take care of them, maintain them, and provide them access to more complex ways of being when they are ready to move. One of the great ethical questions of the last century has been how much to tamper with Level 1 cultures when they are discovered in the hidden places on Earth. Usually, missionaries have made the decision to intervene. However, there are still a few pockets where Level 1 exists in peaceful isolation. Whether to forcibly "advance" them or protect them from external complications that would destroy a balanced well-functioning Level 1 is a tough call. People living in a Level 1 way are not necessarily stupid. On the contrary, they may be able to access natural intelligences misplaced long ago by "civilization."

The homeless in America are not operating at Level 1, but they may at times behave as Level 1s. Behaviorally, Level 1 problems are very real on the street. But, with rare exceptions, homeless people access the higher levels of brain equipment to resolve their situation. Thinking and acting to survive are two different things. That's why the homelessness problem is so tragic — high level thinking wasted on lowest level problems. Many of the homeless have creatively figured out ways to survive.

Homo sapiens began as Level 1s and every one of us begins here. Most of us move to Level 2s as we become toddlers — up the stairs, through various transition steps, to the next landing. Level 1 problems are no less important, but the energy spent solving them drops as more complex Level 2 equipment is brought to bear. A new layer is painted on and a new view of the world is now possible. As our physiological needs are taken care of, we begin to look around, search, and explore our environment. Most people, in a civilized country, begin to move into Level 2 around two to six years of age; however, in developing countries, adults may be caught in a Level 2 environment and their brain continues to function at Level 2.

Level 2: Tribalistic

The Level 2 person begins to realize that as an individual being, I am distinct from others and distinct from the external world, yet dependent on others to resolve Level 1 problems. There is excess energy for looking at the environment and things that happen to other people. Most of it doesn't make a lot of sense, and people find safety in numbers. Thus, the Level 2 is referred to as Tribalistic.

People like things to make sense, and the first way we try to rationalize the world is through magic. We see things happen and attribute events to mystical, anthropomorphized forces — consciousnesses superior to us that want to mess with us. Level 2 conditions are full of superstition and spirits. If Level 2 equipment is operating, it feels safer to hold hands and huddle together. The Communal/Collective is stronger than the lone individual.

Another good word for Level 2 is "animistic." This is the view that objects are possessed of life force; that everything is alive. There are spirits of the water, moon, trees, and seasons. Each spot along the river has a name and a myth, though the river itself might not. Groups at Level 2 often think of themselves as "the people"; others are unknown, rarely encountered, kept at a distance, or seen as enemies. Separateness tightens the group.

Level 2 people are basically passive, though they will readily use force if threatened. They live a life that is strongly defended, but not understood. Tradition and ritualistic thinking provide a means of safety. Magic is ingrained and greatly influences how Tribalistic people behave. Omens, signs, dreams, and interpretations from the shaman determine what is and is not done. Other authority figures, such as chieftains (parents, spouses, teachers, coaches, bosses, police, ministers, etc.) can exert great influence.

There is often a richly developed spirit world in which ancestors and various deities reside. Great power over natural events, birth and death, illness and prosperity, is attributed to them. This mystical realm permeates the lives of Level 2 thinkers, keeping past and present entwined. It can be quite elaborate, with myths and an oral tradition extending into a timeless past. It can also be quite sophisticated, with highly effective "folk" medicines, construction principles, and harmonious environmental awareness.

People centered at Level 2 are quite capable of productive work, so long as it doesn't clash with superstitions or the magical beliefs that so engage their thinking. Though their classical constructions are largely in ruins, there is a rich history of Level 2 achievements. There are still many places on Earth where Level 2 thinking is predominant in large populations, including Indonesia, Tibet, the Andean highlands, Aboriginal Australia, and parts of Central Africa.

We said earlier that everyone reading this book has passed through Level 2. Don't infer that to mean that every reader has abandoned it. Most of us retain our superstitions, sentimentalities, souvenirs, and relics of fantasy surrendered to "the real world." Many of us would be much healthier if we could regain some of the imaginativeness and sense of belonging that so typifies the Level 2 thinking.

Tribalistic adults can work and be managed. In the United States, they may be found in unskilled or semiskilled jobs. People whose thinking is centered around Level 2 prefer jobs that are routine and fairly repetitive. Good, effective managers are directive and available to give immediate feedback as to whether the job is being done well or not so well. It is important to re-emphasize that feedback should be immediate. Ensuring feelings of safety and security is important, as fear contaminates production.

The manager also must see that the Level 2 individual is provided a good model to emulate, for learning comes through repetition, imitation, and modeling. It's a major mistake for management to be too verbal with extensive explanations for what to do. Extensive written instructions are even worse. Level 2s learn best by doing; they acquire skills by imitating a model. Foremen and straw-bosses who are "in the trenches" with their personnel make good managers. Though it was forgotten too often during the Vietnam era, the military has historically understood this well.

Most normal children between the ages of 2 and 6 exhibit a lot of Level 2 thinking. That's when it peaks in the developmental process, with the awakening of Level 2 thinking in response to Level 2 environmental problems — awareness of threats/safety, socialization, sharing, questions about everything.

In a preschool program, we wanted to demonstrate the effects of modeling vs. verbal explanations. We took two groups of 4-and 5-year-olds and taught them to put a napkin in their laps at lunch. One group was identified as "verbal." Those children were told the purpose of the napkin and why it was to be placed in one's lap prior to eating. The teacher demonstrated how to do it, and all children who placed napkins in their laps got verbal praise for doing so. The other group was identified as "model." Those children were told nothing. They arrived and were seated at the lunch table as usual. The teacher rapped on the table with her knuckles to get their attention and, as they watched, the teacher smiled and dramatically picked up the napkin and placed it in her lap. When one of the children followed her example, she turned to the child and said, "I like the way Mary has her napkin in her lap." Immediately, all the children put the napkins in their laps. By the fourth day, all the children in the model group were placing their napkins in their laps as they sat down at the lunch table, prior to the teacher putting the napkin in her lap. Also the napkin-in-lap behavior continued for the rest of the school year. It appeared the children had not only learned to put napkins in their laps, but they became habituated to doing it. After two months, fewer than half the children in the verbal group were putting the napkins in their laps without being told. Admittedly, this delayed behavior could be a function of how the children were verbally instructed, but I am convinced that many Level 2 children learn best by physically doing the task and that learning is facilitated through imitation. (For more information on this study and others, see *Head Start: A Tragicomedy With Epilogue*, by Payne, Mercer, Payne, and Davison).

An 18-year-old child with mental retardation wouldn't hang up his coat when he returned from school. He was functioning primarily at Level 2. For 18 years he had been told, yelled at, talked to, explained to, over and over, and rewarded for hanging up his coat when he came home from school. For 18 years, it hadn't worked. He was not being defiant; he just couldn't remember to hang up his coat. The mother was instructed to put a coat on, hide behind the door, and, as Jimmy came in, jump out and say "Jimmy, I'm glad you're home. Now watch mother." Then the mother would hang her coat up and offer Jimmy a hanger. Jimmy would hang up his coat. After a week, the mother would still appear from behind the door, but would hand Jimmy a hanger and have him hang his coat up before she hung hers up. Next, Jimmy began getting his own hanger as his mother just waited. Finally, Jimmy was hanging his coat up without hint or prompting from his mother. The amazing thing was that this continued. It was apparent that Jimmy had learned and become habituated to hanging up his coat. (Other examples may be found in *Strategies for Teaching Learners with Special Needs*, by Polloway, Patton, Payne, and Payne.)

The power of **PeopleWise® Motivation** is that when we understand how another person thinks — get into another person's head, so to speak — we not only understand that person better, but we can help that person. We're not playing games with them, manipulating them to serve our ends. We're facilitating them to be as effective as they can be, to climb the stairs of life as far as their potential will allow. **PeopleWise® Motivation** lets us pick and choose the most appropriate action because we look beyond who the person is and what the person does and we deal with them brain-to-brain.

Years ago in a community action program, one of the employees was convinced a coworker was a witch and, worse, was making her "need to pee." The coworker would hide and jump out and scare the employee, causing her to run to the bathroom. I tried to explain to the "victim" that there was no such thing as a witch. I pleaded with her to understand. I reasoned with her. I tried separating the two employees, but it did no good since the office was fairly small and they'd end up together some time during the day.

I tried talking to the self-proclaimed "witch." I pleaded. I threatened. She would agree to stop playing her games, but pretty soon she'd be up to her old shenanigans again. Practicing good bureaucratic management at the time, I sent her up before a disciplinary committee for actions and possible termination. Three different times the committee found no grounds for action. Accusations of witchcraft don't stand up well against Civil Service rules, and not being a very nice person isn't sufficient, either.

After three years, as I was leaving the program and moving on, I had a last-minute conference with the victimized employee to try to explain, one final time, that her coworker was not a witch. The victim listened intently as I explained about the coworker's somewhat warped personality, about witchcraft, and anything else I could think of. When I finished, she responded very simply, "If she's not a witch, how come when she is near me I have to pee?" I didn't have the answer. She left the meeting thinking the coworker was a witch; I left thinking the poor victim was a stupid, incompetent, misguided fool. After studying Graves and becoming **PeopleWise®** some years later, I realized that the employee wasn't stupid or incompetent or even misguided. Truth is, she was very smart, was outstanding in her work as a teacher's aide, and wasn't misguided at all. She was well adjusted in her world, and her thinking was consistent with it. Problem was, I mismanaged her.

She was living a Level 2 life and I was trying to impose inappropriate solutions on her. I could have reasoned with her for years about witches and not changed her mind a whit. My logic wasn't hers. She'd have to move to a different Level before she could forget about magic and spells. She was an effective person and did an excellent job working with, surprise, Level 2 children. She learned through imitation and modeling, just as the young children did. It was a simple matter to teach this victimized teacher's aide all the songs, finger plays, dances, and activities the children were to do and then place her in a classroom to function as the model for the children to follow. The trouble was, I never even thought of how to utilize her thinking and her skills with her job, that is, functioning as a model for young children. All I could offer was well-intentioned, but useless, verbiage. Still, looking back on that situation, I realize my incompetence and how misguided and how stupid I was. If only I'd understood **PeopleWise® Motivation** then, I might be a warlock today.

Most people at Level 2 are young children who learn through modeling and imitation, but sooner or later they begin to recognize that some people are not like themselves. They begin to question the power of magic, the omniscience of the wise-ones, and the value of all the traditions. They question authority. They look around and see other people who have more than they do, who are treated as more important, and they wish to be like them. A few will remain satisfied at Level 2; some will have reached the limits of their capacities there; but most will begin climbing up the staircase to the next landing, the next Level: 3 — Egocentric.

CHAPTER NINE

THE VIOLENT STEP THREE

The Level 3 brain equipment is survivalistic, raw, and impulsive. This Level is characterized by fierce competitiveness, aggressiveness, and an "eye-for-an-eye" morality. Power is revered, weakness squashed. It is violent.

It's important to realize that guilt does not exist in the Level 3 brain. There will be fear of shame and loss of face, but guilt hasn't yet emerged. That's both liberating and frightening. It means the person has tremendous degrees of freedom — "if it feels good, do it" — but lacks the ability to think consequentially. Threats of punishment mean little, and only immediate rewards are particularly significant.

Level 3: Egocentric

The Level 3 Egocentric thinker insists that winners in the fight for survival deserve the spoils of their victories. Losers are relegated to submissive subservience. Because thinking is so focused within the self and self's interest, it is commonplace that the powerful individual has the inalienable right to authoritarian control over the lesser ones, the "have-nots." It's also noteworthy that the exploited losers generally hold the same values as their oppressors, but are reduced to a miserable life of trying to beat the system.

In 1970, Graves discussed Level 3 Existence as follows:

> It is a world driven by man's lusts and is seemingly noteworthy for its lack of a "moral sense." But this is an error, for at this level where man is led to value the ruthless use of power, unconscionably daring deeds, impulsive action, volatile emotionality, the greatest risk, morality is ruthlessness ... This is not an attractive value system from other frames of reference, but for all the negative aspects, it is a giant step forward. Some will, in their pursuit of power, tame the mighty river, provide the leisure for beginning intellectual effort, build cities ...

After studying under Graves' tutorage, I became curious as to what really motivated Level 3s. Graves had gathered some data from juveniles and a few prisoners, but found it quite difficult to collect a lot of data on 3s. "Oh, boy. They told me where to go and just what to do when I got there," he once remarked. I decided to study successful adult Level 3 thinkers. I settled on over-the-road truckers. Although not all truckers function at Level 3, many do, so this was a good place to start.

I decided to interview drivers at truck stops along the Pennsylvania Turnpike. Needless to say, this was a research project I'll never forget. If you have ever eaten in a real truck-stop restaurant, you know that most have sections set aside for Professional Truck Drivers Only. Although this seems a bit discriminatory, I needn't discuss the legal ramifications right now. Suffice it to say, these prestigiously reserved areas are sociological artifacts — truck drivers like to be around other truck drivers, people who understand diesel and weights and CBs, not pesky 4-wheeler types.

I sat in this hallowed ground, although I was clearly 14 wheels shy of the norm. After being given the cold shoulder and actually asked to sit in another section — the "Everybody Else" part — I worked myself up to an emotional pitch and insisted that someone in the trucking profession talk with me. I was escorted outside by two guys who made their disinterest in psychological research quite clear.

Being of unsound mind and body, I barged back in and proceeded to tell my escorts that I was damned mad at the bum's rush and that I only wanted to talk to a group of truckers to find out what motivated them to help a group of high school kids with problems and that ...

A large hand grabbed my shoulder and physically seated me beside one of the truckers — slam — with the other sitting across the booth. The one across asked, "Just what the hell do you want?" I could tell, I was softening them up.

"First, how do you know I'm not a trucker?" I asked.

The two looked at one another and laughed. The one beside me said, "Your belt buckle gives you away."

I looked down at my Bill Blass buckle and asked what I thought was an intelligent question, "So what's wrong with my buckle?"

"Hell, that's no buckle. This here's a belt buckle." Both truckers stood up, put their thumbs inside their jeans, and proudly displayed buckles that made mine look like a wimp. They went on to make fun of the tassels on my loafers. I learned that you don't put tassels on boots.

I asked why most of the truckers were wearing boots, anyway. They were riding inside truck cabs, not on horseback, after all. My remark drew a sneer from an adjoining booth and a reminder. "Boots are good for kicking tires ... and other things ... if you get my meaning ..." I did. But then the truckers eventually began to help.

As I collected information on what truckers liked and disliked I discovered that almost every one who was predominantly functioning at Level 3 had disliked school and many of them had never finished high school. As I observed the buying and eating habits of the Level 3 truckers, I found they ate the same things in the same way and their buying tastes were similar. (Every self-respecting truck stop also has a general store.)

The largest-selling piece of jewelry along the turnpike was a woman's necklace with the word "BITCH" prominently displayed, either inscribed or spelled out in rhinestones. How would a woman who'd like wearing such a necklace be thinking? In a Level 3 way, that's how. By the way, you'll find the same piece selling well in Ft. Worth, and Newark, and the tougher parts of L.A. The life of a long-haul trucker is hard. The work is stressful, the money is always tight, and home is often a long way off. It takes strong people to survive and keep on truckin', to keep families intact, and to win against weather and the road.

I found similar eating habits and buying tastes later when I began to study professional football players. Again, I was interested in what motivated players with thinking centered around Level 3. I found one Egocentric interior lineman who could psych himself up by listening to "Eye of the Tiger" prior to going on the field. Another played with greater intensity after placing a picture of General Patton in his locker and putting four stars inside his helmet. He plays "with reckless abandon when he has his four-star helmet on," one of the coaches recalled.

The most unusual motivational finding was with a linebacker who was obsessed with collecting German war relics. He was well read on tanks and artillery of both world wars and had a scrapbook full of pictures. He enjoyed building models of tanks and other military vehicles.

During a counseling session he was asked what really turned him on, what really motivated him, what psyched him up. For a while he couldn't think of anything in particular. But then he mentioned that sometimes when he couldn't sleep, he'd go to his study, look at his scrapbooks, and even put on a German helmet and march around the house. He confessed that with the helmet on, he felt stronger, more powerful — it got his blood moving.

As we discussed the situation, I could tell this helmet business really did something to him psychologically. We explored what it would be like if he were allowed to scrimmage with the German helmet on, in place of his regular football headgear. As we talked, he began to get excited. With permission from the coaches and the front office, we prepared for our first German helmet experimental scrimmage.

The day was unforgettable. He reported to practice early. As he got taped and suited up, he displayed determination and intensity in every movement. As the other players came in, they joked and carried on as usual. Then, in the middle of it all, the Level 3 linebacker, now completely ready except for his helmet, took the black German helmet from his locker, looked at it, polished the top and put it on. As if in a trance, he moved to the full-length mirror at the end of the locker room and stared at himself in admiration. He was almost hyper-ventilating. The other players looked at him incredulously as he sprinted outside.

After leaving, one of the other players asked, "What the heck is this all about?" I explained that we were trying to determine what effect the German helmet would have on motivation.

As everyone lined up for calisthenics and wind sprints, it was obvious that this linebacker was in another world. He was quicker, faster, stronger. You could hear his breathing 25 yards away.

During scrimmage, on the first play, the ball went to the halfback. The offensive line had made a hole big enough to drive a semi through, except that the Level 3 linebacker was in the middle with Hunnish fire in his eyes. The halfback, seeing this human gorilla, momentarily slowed down. At that hesitation, the linebacker shot forward and flattened him so viciously that the halfback's helmet flew off.

In the next plays, the Level 3 linebacker was wild. He was all over the field, in on every tackle. Finally, the quarterback came over to the sidelines. After a bit of discussion with the coaches, it was decided that we'd gone too far and that the German helmet had to go. Later we placed decals of swastikas on the inside of his football helmet, causing a similar effect. While the imagery was personally offensive to us, it was highly motivating to this Level 3 player. Without apparent guilt or concern with what the Nazi symbols represented to many people, he found it thrilling.

PeopleWise® Motivation often means walking a mile in someone else's shoes, even though they may smell a bit rank.

After experiencing the dramatic effect of the German helmet, I wondered what would happen if we used a similar technique with juvenile offenders to motivate them to change their behavior. I was working with six junior high school students who had been identified as potential prison candidates. They'd already had run-ins with the police, all hated school, and all came from rough family backgrounds. I wanted to apply what I'd learned from the truckers and the football players.

Before going into detail, let's review what Level 3 thinking students are like. Any teacher can spot them a mile away. The student, regardless of age, looks meaner, dresses meaner, acts meaner, smells meaner, and is meaner than the non-Level 3 classmates. Whether the students are male or female, they tend to be trouble-makers, frequently fighting or picking on someone. To assist the students in developing self-control and self-discipline, they are subjected to counseling, warnings, yelling-ats, threats, visits to the principal, punishment, and eventually expulsion.

Their homes are likely to be full of Level 3 conditions, with little reliable structure or reason to feel safe and secure — not much to bring order to disorderly thinking or discipline to take into school. The belief in the Level 3 home is that you must fight for everything and that life is full of adversaries. The family car may have a bumper sticker like the one I saw recently: "My Kid Beat Up Your Honor Student." Many of these kids have experienced killings, cuttings, drugs, and violence very early in life. Those experiences actuate brain equipment that can deal with such traumas. That doesn't mean the kids will perpetuate that lifestyle, but it becomes part of "normal" living.

One of the key elements of **PeopleWise® Motivation** insists that before anything positive can happen in a teaching, counseling, managing, or motivational relationship, the teacher, counselor, manager, or motivator must accept individuals for what they are, and every endeavor must start where they are. So we have two lessons: (a) If you plan to help anyone you must first accept people as they are psychologically and (b) You must start working with them where they are psychologically. In other words, you've got to get in their minds in order to work brain-to-brain.

That does not mean condoning what individuals do, only accepting their right to be who they are. People tend to do what they believe should or must be done, and most often we will not be consulted. They behave in accordance with the problems in the environment that confront them and the mental equipment they have available. Human behavior is logically consistent unless the person is mentally ill. So, we start where people psychologically are, recognizing that they function quite "normally" at their various Levels. We best motivate from their mental perspective, from their frame of reference, from their vision of life, from their picture.

I was once talking with a Level 3 junior high student and, during the conversation, mentioned that I liked his leather coat and asked to try it on. He looked somewhat puzzled, but allowed it. Even though it was a bit small, the remark was made how good the coat felt. "You know, when I have this coat on I feel different."

He looked a little surprised and said, "You know, so do I."

"How do you feel different?"

"When I put my coat on it makes me feel more powerful, stronger. It makes me proud. You know, I live in a very rough section of town and we have a lot of fights. This coat protects me."

Later, I admired his combat boots and his reply was, "You know, these boots are like having a motorcycle."

"What do you mean, a motorcycle?"

"Well, I can be walking down the sidewalk when it's raining cats and dogs and if I want I can cut through yards, alleys, puddles. I can go anywhere I feel like in these boots."

This tough little guy was a Walter Mitty. He saw himself as a knight in leather armor, riding a mythical motorcycle down the mean streets of his neighborhood. Few adults would ever compliment him on his coat, and probably none would mention his boots. But he was obviously proud of his coat and boots. They meant something important to him and they motivated him.

There are many articles in professional journals about aggressive children wearing coats and jackets to school and never taking them off. Experiments have been run on getting students to remove coats in "appropriate" circumstances. There are many hypotheses about the jacket phenomenon: Coats are means of security; they provide group/gang identity; kids with holes in their shirts wear jackets to hide them and save face; a coat can mask embarrassing body odor.

My experience is that Level 3 students like wearing shirts with "character," whether that means holes or not. They dislike shiny new clothes that non-Level 3s might approve of; they want to stand apart from the group. They like potent smells and eschew clean gym clothes.

When Level 3 thinking becomes extreme, they'll hurt people for shoes and mug people for their jackets. These apparently symbolic possessions take on huge significance in the Egocentric mind. Educators and politicians bemoan the deterioration of values among inner-city youth. We need to understand that the problem is deeper than simply what kids believe; it's how they think and the ways their brains function. When the Level 3 is in command, death is no big deal and what happens to others is incidental. Consciousness is locked into the egocentric self.

If we are to help people at the Level 3 through better management, education, and motivation, we must accept who they are and try to understand how they think and see themselves. We've got to start from where they are, not from where we want them to be. If we seriously set out to teach, counsel, manage, or motivate such individuals, the worst thing we can initially do is to force the literal or symbolic removal of their coats or imply that we don't approve of who they are. Once we've accepted who the individuals are, it's time to start work.

In the project with six Level 3 junior high school students, we hired a karate teacher to come to the school twice a week and give them lessons in the martial arts. The instructor was an oriental woman in her mid-thirties who weighed less than the students. Each lesson lasted less than an hour.

Prior to the first session, we filled her in on the histories of the six tough kids and warned her about their attitudes. She said she could handle it, no problem, and asked only that we let her work her own way.

On the first day she arrived in sandals and a karate outfit, carrying three bricks. None of the students paid any attention. She put two of the bricks down beside the door and quickly placed the third on the teacher's desk. She walked back to the door and slipped off her sandals, putting them right beside the bricks on the floor. She turned around and strode directly back to the desk. She bowed slowly, with great dignity, to the brick. Then she stepped back and crouched into an attack position. This tiny woman shifted laterally a couple of times, let out a shriek, arched into the air and brought her bare heel down onto the brick, splitting it cleanly in half.

All the kids looked at her with their eyes wide open. She calmly turned to the group and announced, "I like aggression; I like violence; and I like fighting. By the time I am through with you this year, each one of you will be able to break a brick with your heel just like I did." She then walked to the door, slipped on her sandals, and left. Talk about getting someone's attention!

The amazing thing was that for the rest of the year, this diminutive lady never had to raise her voice, never had any discipline problems, never had to threaten anyone. She had the respect of these tough kids and knew they needed respect in return. The karate instructor understood Level 3 thinking, she accepted it as how these kids saw the world, and she began working with them from the Level 3.

Later in the year we decided to use the lesson from the line-backer and try military helmets. We got one for each of the students with the word "READING" stenciled on it. We told them that every time they went to reading class they were to wear their helmets because going to reading was like going to war. We told them we knew reading was difficult for them, would probably always be difficult, and if they were to succeed at it they'd have to psych themselves up. The helmets were to symbolize power, hardship, and determination. As you might guess, when they wore the helmets the students tried harder, made reading gains, and stayed at the task longer.

One of the major lessons of **PeopleWise® Motivation** is that when you accept people as they are and you begin at their psychological levels, they trust you more and will work harder and enjoy it. Even more significantly, they may begin to change themselves. You can never guarantee that change will occur, but you can virtually be sure it won't if you try to manage from levels too far apart from the person or group. **PeopleWise® Motivation** requires that systems be in sync with where people are and adapt to where they can go.

When we taught the Level 3 football players how to motivate themselves through music, decals, helmets, etc., they not only played more intently and aggressively on the field, they got into less trouble in the community. Arrests went down as they learned they were in control of their emotions and could turn the motivational spigot on and off at will. In other words, there was a time to be aggressive and a time not to. The players learned how to tell the difference and developed the skills to behave appropriately to time and place. They developed healthier ways to exhibit their Level 3 urges — they didn't abandon them. Prior to the motivational training, the Level 3 players actually believed they couldn't control their aggressiveness — it was just in them — "the devil made me do it" sort of thing.

The six tough junior high school kids showed obvious academic gains over the year. They, too, seemed to learn when to fight and when not to. They found ways to control their Level 3 impulsivity without abandoning their sense of self. About halfway through the year, after the students began to trust us and their own abilities, we taught a lesson on appropriate dress. The ones who had insisted on wearing their jackets in class began to hang them in the closet while in school. It showed confidence in us, in themselves, and in the other students. All this was accomplished without harassment, reprimand, or threat.

The lesson worked because a solid base of trust was established, mutual respect was operating, and the kids believed we really were interested in their welfare. After that year, they had significantly fewer run-ins with the law and performed better in school. None has gone to jail or even gotten into any real trouble in the years since the program was completed. **PeopleWise® Motivation** works, both in the short run as well as in the long run.

People do better when they are motivated appropriately. Once again, revise the Golden Rule: Do not treat others the way you want to be treated, but the way they themselves want to be treated. People function at different Levels and we will make more meaningful strides in education, management, and law enforcement when we accept the basic premise that different people have different expectations of how they should be treated. The fact is people's brains fire differently.

A large number of people exist primarily at this level. Many third-world nations are just passing out of Level 3 governmental structures. America's cities are showing an increase in Level 3 thinking, particularly among youth. Crime statistics and generally uncivilized behavior increasing on freeways tend to bear this out.

As a society, we do not seem willing or able to come to grips with the situation, largely because decision makers operating from much higher levels still refuse to accept that people are functioning at the Level 3 and must be dealt with according to its rules. The idea that some brains may peak at Level 3 just drives "do-gooders" nuts. At the same time, the unwillingness of many helpers to "stoop to their level" precludes effective intervention with those who have greater potential. Many people just wring their hands at the idea of coming into contact with Level 3s. They are not **PeopleWise®**.

Level 3s can be managed, but most managers can't handle more than three at once. And everybody doesn't have the skills — cops call it "presence" — but too many teachers, bosses, and parents give up before applying the correct tools. Level 3 people have high energy levels — often misdirected — which can be focused toward constructive ends. If handled improperly, though, they will use ruthless, guilt-free force to exploit a business, a school, a community, or their peers for their own Egocentric needs.

Level 3 thinkers are best managed in an authoritarian manner. Managers must "out-power" the person into taking directions and guidance. They must not undercut or shame, however, as this only triggers a cycle of vengeance and retribution. Moderated by reasonable compassion and sensitivity (but never weakness or uncertainty), this exploitative authoritarian style can get productive work. Level 3 operators will walk all over a perceived patsy and rebel if they sense they're being maneuvered. The more action, the better; but it must be kept in check.

As Level 3 thinkers go along fighting, being rough, "taking nothing off nobody," and doing whatever feels good, some, if not most, suddenly wake up and realize a person can get killed doing that stuff. Mortality begins to register. A new set of problems begins to take shape — the meaning of life, dealing with consequences of one's actions, awareness of other people and their rights — that activates the Level 4 equipment and moves the person to Level 4 thinking.

CHAPTER TEN

HUMANKIND GIANT STEPS FOUR AND FIVE

Self-sacrifice is the order of the day. The quest for stability and the desire of hope for an unknown future structure this thinking. Whether based on religion or some other organizing principle, there's usually belief in a master plan, a division of people into classes, punishment for transgressions and reward for righteous deeds, some day. Because guilt is a key factor in Level 4 thinking, fault-finding and maintaining discipline occupy lots of energy. Level 4 thinking is absolutist thinking.

Level 4: Absolutist

The values of hard work, self-sacrifice, commitment, dutifulness, and getting ahead by putting ones shoulder to the wheel and nose to the grindstone fit the Level 4 mindset quite well. One is expected to make the most of who one was meant to be, to know and keep one's rightful place, and not to make waves. The call to support those in authority rings out. Symbols like flags and sacred places are important. Whereas Level 2 has its shaman and medicine man, Level 4 reveres its high priests, the divine right of monarchs, and the chain of command.

The Level 4 family is "traditional" because of a linkage between past and future. Life often centers around children and grandchildren. Continuity of generations brings stability and a way to pass life on. The family unit is also the support system for its members, taking care of its own and instilling responsibility. Ceremonies like christenings, weddings, bar mitzvahs, and quinzinellas mark life's transitions.

When Level 4 thinking is applied to work, we ordinarily think of the Puritan work ethic. Respect abounds for those who work long, hard, dutiful hours, who work their way up, and who earn what they've got through the honest sweat of their brows. Everybody must pay the price. The 25-year pin, the gold watch, and the retirement banquet are important and significant.

Yet it's also possible to establish a Level 4 tradition of non-work. The welfare cycle sometimes locks families into a pattern that extends across generations as well. Children learn what's right, normal, and acceptable by living it. There can be a powerful fatalism in Level 4, a resignation to what seems ordained to be.

When dealing with Level 4 thinkers, it's important to recognize the importance of lists, rules, punctuality, job descriptions, rank, and authority. Things are best done in sequence, first things first. Too many variables lead to confusion of the mind.

Loyalty to group, company, or cause is characteristic of Level 4. Honor and devotion help Level 4 organizations endure in adversity. They want to last forever. This way of thinking ran the machines of the Industrial Revolution, brought "civilization" to the American frontier, and still populates the armies of the world. Though sometimes exploited by unscrupulous con-artists or misled by skillful demagogues, people operating at Level 4 get satisfaction out of sacrificing for their companies, families, or nations.

Learning occurs from respected higher authority figures. Whereas Level 3s need a steady stream of rewards, Level 4 thinkers respond to punishment. They fear failure and feel guilt when letting down family, group, or standards. Thus, most Level 4 legal systems are based in "Thou shalt nots" and corresponding penalties, not rewards or incentives for being good.

Cookbook education works at Level 4. Tell it like it is; put it down in logical steps to be followed; and evaluate it right or wrong. People operating at this Level prefer practical things to abstract theory, matter-of-fact approaches to ambiguity or doubt. Tight structure, linear sequences, regimentation, and limits are necessary. Much of traditional education was and is based on precisely this model. However, if Level 4 thinking has not yet turned on in the students' brains, then learning will not likely occur through traditional means. Level 4 teaching is effective with Level 4 learners. If they're still predominantly in Level 3, everybody's wasting time until they get in sync.

When teaching at the university, I appeal to Level 4 students by providing a tidily structured outline of the lectures. It further helps when I put the same outline on an overhead projector or project it electronically using PowerPoint. It's best to proceed from the beginning right through to the end according to the written plan.

This really helps the Level 4 students to feel like they're learning. They can follow along visually and take notes on the handout. When I want to do a bit of game playing, and at the same time demonstrate a point, I proceed through the lecture in the usual fashion I-A, B, C, then II-A, B, C, then III-A. I skip III-B and go right to C. Invariably, a student will raise a hand and ask, "But what about III-B?"

I look puzzled, fumble with notes, glance at the screen, and then say, "Oh, don't worry about III-B. That's a typographical error and shouldn't be on this outline anyway." The really compulsive Level 4s grab their erasers and aggressively try to erase III-B out of existence, sometimes rubbing a hole right through the paper. The non-Level 4s merely check off III-B, relabel III-C, or just don't worry about it.

These Level 4 students are telling us, "I learn best when there are no surprises. I prefer to stay in Holiday Inns where there are no surprises. I learn best from a lock-step method." Level 4 learners like to know the absolute truth.

Level 4s are best managed through directiveness and prescribed rules and procedures. They are most productive and happiest under such a regime. Fairness, equity, and consistency are important and should be practiced "by the book." A work environment that is highly ordered, structured, and organized fits just right. Managers must prescribe and enforce the rules. The benevolent autocrat who is on the one hand firm, directive, and authoritative and, on the other, warm, fair, straight-arrow, and philanthropic is right in sync.

Problems arise when you have two pure Level 4 groups with different books from different viewpoints. Absolutistic thinking engenders strong us/them feelings with friends and foes, truth and blasphemy, good and evil clearly delineated. Sometimes, all that is exchanged are derogatory glances. When 4-on-4 escalates, though, conflicts and ongoing warfare result — racial, political, religious, or any combination thereof.

An important part of the Level 4 world view is respect for authority figures. Those in authority are expected to play the part — to look, dress, and act appropriately. Insignia of rank or "proper business attire" is the visual cue that the person understands the role. Here is an example of some 4-ness in me as to the importance of looking, acting, and dressing the part of a Level 4.

I once had to fly to a small town to give a lecture. For the last leg, I transferred to a little 8-seat aircraft. I'd never been in a plane this small before. As I got in and buckled up, I looked forward and found there was no bulkhead. The pilot's seats and instrument panel with all its gauges and gadgets were right there, out in plain sight. It looked very complex and for a second or two I was frightened.

When the lump in my throat settled, I looked around and found I was the only passenger. The pilot boarded, introduced himself as "Jerry," and clumsily settled into the left seat. He comfortingly advised me, "Don't worry. This won't take long. We'll be up and down before you know it."

Although I have to fly a lot on large commercial airlines, I thought this was unique, a little too unique. What really bothered me was that "Jerry" wasn't in a uniform. He was wearing a hunting jacket and baseball cap with a patch on the cap that said, "Pilots get high in the sky." It was just too much for me. I unbuckled my seat belt, told "Jerry" there'd been a change in plans, and deplaned.

For all I know, he may have been an excellent pilot and it might have been a fine flight. But when I pay the prices they charge to fly today, I want a pilot in a uniform I can trust. I prefer to hand my life over to somebody who conforms to my Level 4 expectations. The bus ride was excellent, by the way. The driver was wearing a well-pressed uniform and a proper sort of cap.

Hard work, dedication, and loyalty satisfy Level 4s. These people find answers to their questions about what life means, build faith in what is to come, and come to believe in some purpose greater than themselves. Then comes the shift. Once the Level 4 problems are reasonably under control, there is time to think about the here-and-now.

Some Level 4s come to realize that not everybody lives in the same way. They see that others have things they don't. Some people seem to have nicer things and live easier lives.

They've kept the faith, but what is it getting them? They've lived the righteous existence, but where's the payoff? They've supported the one true way, but those who believe otherwise are prospering, not being punished. The idea that "the" way may only be "a" way starts to emerge. Doubt about the infallibility of higher authority begins to appear. The notion that there are possibilities to do better for those who will take some risks is introduced into their thinking. The individual begins to reassert dominance as the collective backs down and, for some, the move to Level 5 is on.

Again, some people will stop at Level 4. They may find deep satisfaction in the unending struggle to lead the "good" life. Or they may not have access to Level 5 thinking. In other words, their brain continues to fire at the Level 4. If that's the case, no amount of training will turn the person into a Level 5. No experience will break down the absolutist wall. And no decent person will try to force the shift on people who are satisfied, productive, and happy as they are.

Level 5: Materialist

When people move into Level 5, they begin to manage their guilt. As the individual, expressive self begins to predominate again, they conclude that sheer hard work and perseverance don't necessarily win. And winning is what Level 5 living is all about. Why not experience "the good life," here and now? Why not find ways to understand the Level 4 system so well it can be controlled for one's personal advantage? Rather than dutiful obedience, strategic thinking takes over.

The Level 5 thinker sees options, alternatives, and possibilities all around. Perhaps someone was promoted because of political connections or being "in the right place at the right time" instead of earning it. Or, maybe the person actually did know more, was smarter, and could handle greater complexity. At Level 5, there's advantage in working smarter rather than just harder, and there's usually a plan for getting ahead.

Whereas Level 4's categorical thinking resists change, a Level 5 relishes it. Novelty — the new-and-improved — plays right into the goal of making life even better. This leads to competitiveness, even aggressiveness. Unlike Level 3, the aggression is tempered with some guilt and an awareness of Level 4's rules. But Level 5 still plays to win. Whether at athletics, love, or games, the aim is always to come out #1. In case of a loss, it's "Let's make it two out of three."

When the Level 5 mind is activated, the person starts thinking in cause-and-effect terms — if you do A, B will probably happen. People can cause things to happen, they make their own breaks, and they're responsible for their own destinies. No longer pawns in a pre-ordained chess game of life, the Level 5 thinkers mold, change, and develop the environment to suit the self. They act and proact rather than react or accept.

Accountability is big at Level 5. The individual is responsible for actions. There is no grand design to blame, no celestial scapegoat to predestine failure. Thinking is results-oriented, outcome-based, and evaluative. Nice tries don't count against the cold printout of the bottom line.

Motion-through-space analysis is characteristic of Level 5 thinking. That refers to objectively determining the positioning of a thing relative to others in a given situation. You can observe individuals in the military and immediately tell what rank they hold by dress and decoration.

In a Level 5 business, you can measure someone's importance by observing the office. Beginners with low status are placed in an office pool where they share supplies and equipment with others. Next, they may get a personal space complete with credenza and book shelves. An office overlooking the work pool comes next, then one with a window onto the parking lot. A wooden desk replaces metal, carpet appears, and even a personal secretary. Eventually, a corner office overlooking green space, an adjoining restroom, and conference facilities.

In organizations based in Level 5 assumptions, you know how important persons are by checking out their office. This "motion-through-space" concept explains why Level 5 thinkers want the latest and finest gimmicks — executive toys, luxury cars, and expensive houses. Life is a constant effort to get ahead of the Joneses, to acquire happiness, and to prove self-worth.

Material signs of success are important. In pro sports, Level 5 players are motivated by juicy contracts, opulent lifestyles, and being winners. Schoolboys are motivated by being a somebody and getting special treatment. If a player makes so many tackles or so many touchdowns, Pow!, a decal for the helmet or a star on the locker. As the season goes on, more and more stickers appear. What does this do? For Level 5 thinkers, it maintains interest and helps them work harder and enjoy it at the same time.

You can often spot a young person walking down the hall in a high school wearing a letter jacket. There's usually a symbol identifying the event — football, gymnastics, band, tennis, drill team, baseball, or even debate. Hash-marks represent the number of years and pins may indicate other special achievements. So what's the kid saying if Level 5 is in operation? "I'm important. I'm somebody. I'm a winner that competes and makes things happen." Kids thinking in other Levels might wear the same sweater, but for different reasons — uniformity, acceptance, good luck, etc. At Level 5, if you've got it, you flaunt it.

Both Levels 3 and 5 are concerned with conquering the world and gaining dominion over it. They differ in their methods and motives. Level 3 uses force and power with reckless abandon, without guilt, and with gusto. Level 5 weighs probabilities and rationally approaches the challenge in ways that achieve results without arousing the wrath of others in opposition.

One of the great assets available at the Level 5 is multiplistic thinking — the ability to handle many things at once, keep several irons in the fire, and juggle several deals simultaneously. Thus, the successful 5th Level operator is often a "leader" at many things, enjoying influence and the ability to control events. It is the essence of entrepreneurism and fundamental to capitalism and free-market economies.

You can find Level 5 thinking in all walks of life. What will set it apart is the competitive urge and the drive to expand, grow, get better, and become renewed. Some archetypical nests of Level 5 thinking are big business, the law, cosmetic surgery, real estate, and Wall Street. Its excesses brought down U.S. savings and loans, weakened the automobile and steel industries, and threaten the environment. This thinking has also extended our life expectancies, found ways to feed a growing population, and brought the world into instantaneous contact.

Appropriate motivation for Level 5 is firm but fair autocracy mixed with perks for excellent performance. Economic incentives and end-of-year bonuses sweeten the pot. Level 5s absolutely love merit-pay schemes. Seniority-based hierarchies and no avenues for getting ahead are demotivating factors. Issues need to be handled in an objective fashion with quantifiable data and "the facts." Feelings and group allegiances may be abandoned in the face of harsh "reality." Hard-ball bargaining and "take name and kick tail" approaches fit well, though the kicks may be symbolic — no key to the executive washroom or being uninvited to play golf. Level 5 people like to be "players," VIPs in the game of life, influential and recognized as such. They want to be part of first-class organizations and resent anyone's resting on laurels.

Those thinking in this way respect the mastery of power and the wielding of clout. The need for categories that rise at Level 4 begins to disappear with the turning-on of Level 5 thinking. Lines become flexible and change is possible. Since "the" truth is only "a" truth at this Level, differences can coexist without confusing things. Debate and agreeable disagreements are possible once information is based on probabilities and not sacred doctrine. Error is no longer so threatening, and fallibility can be excused if it doesn't happen more than once.

You've probably already realized that Levels 4 and 5 constitute the core of American thinking. They're the nucleus of "Western" civilization and the foundation for many of the great religions of today's world. Level 4 and 5 thinking have advanced humankind as we know it today.

It's a mistake to lump them together in motivation because there are some important differences in these two ways of thinking. Many are obvious, others more subtle; but responding to them differentially makes the difference between high and low productivity, satisfied or miserable employees, and schools that work or don't. **PeopleWise® Motivation** is crucial at all Levels, but it is particularly important to motivate brain-to-brain at Levels 4 and 5.

When people are operating around Level 4, they prefer a controlled, deliberate, and fairly predictable environment. It doesn't need to be as ritualized as Level 2, but consistency is still important. Things need to be done "right" and by the book. Stability, order, respect for authority, and discipline count big.

The Level 5 is more active and assertive. Because individualism is high, there tends to be more wheeling-and-dealing, deviation from norms and traditions, and experimentation with things that are different. The security that protocol and standardized procedures offer matters less than tangible results. Novelty, flexibility, and dynamism increase along with the belief that "my way is the right way."

While working with a corporation that had a Level 5 general manager and a Level 4 business manager, I really learned the difference between the two ways of thinking. The general manager was a man who enjoyed making things happen. He enjoyed changing things; he liked to get results; and he wanted them fast. He would try out all the latest ideas. He read every new book, article, pamphlet he could get his hands on.

The business manager was a woman who believed her job was to give the organization order and continuity. She was concerned with keeping the boat afloat and stable, not necessarily in winning any races. She preferred things not to change. She valued loyalty to the company and wanted employees who were dependable, punctual, hard-working, and serious.

Now, the general manager also appreciated employees who were all of those things, but what he really wanted were people who got results, who came up with unique and novel approaches to problems, who were bright and quick, and who presented a good image for the company.

The business manager, from her Level 4 perspective, believed the best employees (a) needed to work — they were both hungry and dutiful, (b) shouldn't be too attractive — that implied vanity and meant they would have interests other than their jobs, and (c) weren't overly bright — people who are too sharp quickly become bored in routine tasks and aspire to change things or try to learn more than they need to know.

Of course, the general manager wanted people who were highly intelligent so they could learn everything they could to gain competitive advantage. He was constantly sending someone to school for training or to conferences to scout out the latest tricks. He wanted attractive-looking personnel who dressed well because his Level 5 assumption was that customers patronize organizations with crisp, sharp-looking, desirable people in a classy place. He also thought employees should have enough money to enjoy themselves when they were not working because that would enhance their self-images and would, in turn, improve performance.

These two executives were in constant disagreement. Their philosophies of what made a "good" company were quite different. Fortunately, they were highly intelligent people and both liked and understood one another. That is, while both were convinced of the correctness of their own positions, they were able to consider the other's view without rancor or becoming defensive. They respected each other and were able to learn from each other.

That would not have been possible had they been close-minded — "my way is the only way" — but they were open and receptive to each other. Together, using their different viewpoints as an additive asset and not a subtractive liability, they took a financially troubled company, during a recession, and turned it around to being number one in its region.

You can find compulsiveness in both Levels 4 and 5. Level 4 thinkers are often perfectionistic, accurate, digitized, and focused on standards. The Level 5s get locked into success and winning the game, not details or learning the rules. While 4 is trying to handle guilt and obligations, 5 is comparing achievements and laying plans to get ahead.

When trying to talk with Level 5 operators, you sometimes get "selective listening." They tend only to hear what they want to hear and to remember only the parts that serve their ends. They may conveniently forget those things that don't fit their agendas and genuinely believe their rearranged version is true. When giving instructions, it's often wise to have them repeat what they heard and agree to concrete action. You may even want a witness!

The Level 4 needs precise direction as to what the expectations are and what should be done. You may have to explain things over and over until there is no doubt or uncertainty. A written follow-up (neat, but not gaudy) is generally appropriate. Clear, concise, uncomplicated messages that are free of ambiguity and typographical errors are best.

Level 4 people often have difficulty taking a compliment. Self-deprecation and guilt may be lurking in the background. Compliments mean the most when coming from a respected higher authority or recognized "expert." They are accustomed to fault-finding and blame, but may be pleasantly surprised to be told when things are positive. Level 4 organizations — paper-shuffling bureaucracies, for example — often overlook that. The response of Level 5 thinkers to compliments is more likely, "So what else is new? What did you expect?" or "I know I'm good, why aren't you telling everyone?"

Level 4 is territorial. The Level 3 protects its turf and marks its space with spray paint. Level 4 builds picket fences and resents trespassing. This person lays claim to a particular chair in the classroom, a desk in the office, or a place in line. You'll hear a lot about "my computer," "my stapler," and "my tools." Most possessions have name tags and a prescribed location where they belong. It's most upsetting when a borrowed item is not returned on time.

Those with a large proportion of Level 5 thinking tend to use anything they can get their hands on, whether it's theirs or not. After all, if it's not, it should be. While the Level 5 wants to move and move quickly, Level 4 stands up for the status quo and resists change for fear of risking security.

Level 5 sometimes moves too abruptly, while Level 4 holds back too long. While Level 5 is assuming command, Level 4 is demonstrating loyalty. 5 sets goals and plans strategy; 4 concentrates on the task at hand by doing one thing at a time. Level 4 thinking sees things in terms of black or white, while Level 5 likes dabbling in the grays.

Level 4 learning style is through indoctrination by authority and acceptance of the truth. Benjamin Franklin said, "He that teaches himself hath a fool for a master." As the Level 5 way of thinking is added, people begin to learn through trial-and-error experimentation, simulations, and competitive games; the self is empowered.

Training and education at Level 4 are designed to instill the truth. Learning must be practical and applicable. Horace Mann once wrote, "Education must bring the practice as nearly as possible to the theory." At Level 5, people learn in order to improve and advance. Since truth lies within the individual, good information comes from many sources, not just recognized authorities.

People centered around both Levels 4 and 5 admired Vince Lombardi, but for different reasons. Lombardi advocated the hard work, self-sacrifice, blood, sweat, and tears that feel good to the 4th Level brain. He also insisted on winning — "the only thing" — and the thrill of victory is what stimulates Level 5.

Dr. James S. Payne

Level 4 motivation involves rules, policies, security, custom, order, and punishment. Level 5 is concerned with incentives, rewards, advancement, competitive edge, motion-through-space, data-gathering, and evaluation. As you can see, these two Levels comprise the core of the working population. Difficulties arise when organizations fail to realize that Levels 4 and 5 are not alone. Levels 2 and 3 are very much a part of the population still, and Levels 6, 7, and 8 are gaining ground.

CHAPTER ELEVEN

GLOBAL CONSCIOUSNESS STEPS SIX AND SEVEN

The Level 5 person gets caught up with life in the fast lane, running in the fast track, and playing it fast and loose. Keeping ahead of the Joneses by competing in everything — better house, newer car, higher-achieving kids, more successful career — leads to one of three things. First, the cycle may never stop as the individual strives to catch the elusive golden ring of satisfaction. Second, the person may awaken to the notion that there is something else beyond material possessions, money, prestige, and being number one that may bring happiness after all. Or third, the Level 5 family produces offspring who look at the world from atop the parents' shoulders and say, "Yes, that's well and good, but look at what else there is to life." Sometimes Level 5 parents think those kids have gone nuts; others may recognize that there are many legitimate, but different, ways to see what life's about.

Level 6: Sociocentric

A Level 6 person is interested in affiliation, love, acceptance, and coming to peace with who one is. The very strengths of Level 5 — competitive advantage, self above others, win/lose activities, data analysis, and emphasis on development and growth — tend to isolate the individual. While those whose thinking peaks out at Level 5 may think this is all quite fine, others who have more complex systems waiting for activation do not. They see the emotional component of life as absolutely crucial for a healthy, happy existence. This way of thinking is empathetic and sensitive, self-disclosing and deeply concerned with relationships and making connections with other humans.

Strong Level 4s are at odds with 6s. Level 6 thinking includes spontaneity, loose structure, and permissiveness. Level 6s want harmony and agreement. Consensus and loosely bonded teams in which everybody is a sharing equal are the rule.

You can see how this approach is often antithetical to Level 4s who need structure, sharp lines, and order. Yet they really aren't opposites. Both are communal/collective ways of thinking, subsume the individual in a greater whole, and set up norms for acceptable behavior within the group. Level 4 emerges out of the anarchy and chaos of Level 3, imposing external control to coordinate thinking into a linear pattern. Level 6 rises from the frustration of Level 5, trying to bring community and brotherhood back to the divisive competitiveness of that way of living. Levels 4 and 6 restore order from outside the individual, but there is quite a difference between devout prayers for salvation and mind-expanding group experiences.

Although possessions and ownership of things don't play a big part in Level 6 — that's part of the shift away from 5 — symbolism is important. Posters ("Today is the first day of the rest of your life"), poems (Kahlil Jibran), songs (the Beatles in their metaphysical period), and buttons ("Make Love, Not War") are often part of the Level 6 *milieu*. Crystals, Native American crafts, and African artifacts are also popular. (Level 5 buys them as "collectibles" and investments; Level 6 because of the Karma and vibes they exude. Strong Level 6 thinkers often return artifacts to their "rightful" Level 2 places of origin.)

Movements and social causes attract Level 6 thinkers because of their needs to feel togetherness and the urge to give of the self for higher purpose, to connect beyond the material world. Level 5's most important product is progress; for Level 6, it's people. In the 1960s, a time when Level 6 gained prominence, mind-altering drugs and communal living were popular. The Beatles said it best in their song *Revolution*. "You know, we all want to change the world."

Many graduates of the Level 6 Counter-Culture have moved into computers and the "Information Age." Andrew Fleugelman, editor of the original *Whole Earth Catalog*, remarked that "I hope the establishment realizes it is being revolutionized by decentralizing power through the refinement of computers." Many of the Woodstock alumni are trying to shake up the establishment from within, not through overthrow. While a few leftover hippies remain, the new display of Level 6 thinking is in issues like the environment, world hunger, the homeless, early childhood education, health care, etc.

Other common themes are human rights, social services, and liberation of the oppressed. Though various ways of thinking are attached to these issues, the Level 6 attraction is the "make this a better world for you and me in the here-and-now" motive. That can become the downside for Level 6. In the drive to prove all people are precious, unique, and have worth and goodness, naive 6 pulls down the walls that contain the negative aspects of other ways of thinking. Level 3s are set loose to plunder without consequences; Level 4s are allowed to spew venom and demagoguery; and Level 5s are liberated to profit unmercifully in the name of doing good.

People functioning at Level 6 learn best through observation and involvement with others — study groups, seminar classes, and "hanging-out." The following is a hypothetical case that puts Level 6 thinking in perspective.

A seminar facilitator can really motivate the Level 6s by taking off his tie, dressing casually, and not acting like an authority. For example, at the first session, we join around a table and begin with a remark on "... how lucky we are to be together at the university in a class small enough that we can really get to know each other and learn from each other."

"You know, if we could just tap the knowledge and wisdom at this table we could fill volumes. Each one of us brings knowledge that would stagger the mind of mortal man if we could pool it." This really gets Level 6's attention. "During this semester there'll be no text, nor tests or quizzes. No test can be developed that will measure what we really learn. A standard text, regardless of how well written, would only narrow our thinking and limit our learning. We will choose topics for discussion a week in advance so we can think about them ahead of time. Everyone will be peer-graded based on who they uniquely are."

By this time, Level 6 students think they've died and gone to academic heaven. Unfortunately, graduate classes are rarely made up of people at a single Level. There are always several 4s and, after the preceding spiel, they don't know what to do. When the tie comes off, they wonder what's next. They view the casual dress as sloppy and unprofessional. At the mention of no text or exams, the Level 4 students think, "I knew it. The S.O.B. doesn't know enough to teach. We are just going to sit around all semester, waste time talking, and never learn what's right. This guy's trying to draw a salary and not do anything." Some Level 4s drop the class. One or two go to the Dean (higher authority) to register complaints.

Since friendship, tolerance, and sincerity are important values, Level 6 thinkers do not respond well to threats or traditional individual-oriented rewards like money, prestige, or getting ahead of someone else. Resistance is encountered to directive counseling, authoritarian management, and highly structured, task-oriented work. Level 6 demands that everybody be treated as individuals and rebels at being handled "by the book" or as a number.

Non-directive techniques, involvement, and participation work well in Level 6 groups. Everyone needs to have a say and be part of the collective group. Although the egalitarian style leads to high acceptance for group decisions, it may not produce the best outcomes. Alas, what sometimes occurs in Level 6 organizations is the pooling of ignorance and the refusal to let an individual expert take charge. It often takes a long time to accept that the community is wrong and that sharing is not the only way to live.

Level 6 management tends to be democratic, though more a "sense-of-the-meeting" consensus than a counting of votes. McGregor's Theory Y, Blake and Mouton's 9-1, quality circles, and the participatory management movement are all aimed at appealing to Level 6 thinkers and increasing effectiveness. This approach is not a universally accepted management style; those at Levels 3 through 5 often look at Level 6s as nice but soft, weak, and unrealistic.

Managers high in Level 6 thinking can be effective with Level 6 personnel and even with a few at Level 4, if reciprocal warmth/respect is established. It's tough for a Level 6 to manage Level 3s without back-up, and Level 5s often feel like time's-a-wastin' with all the groupiness and feelings talk. Stars have trouble in a choir.

People thinking at Level 6 are tuned-in to other people, concerned with affect, and anxious to be accepted. In spite of the openness and spontaneity, they sometimes get burned. Someone takes advantage or rips them off. Perhaps they just turn a cheek too often. Eventually, some

Level 6s get stymied and think, "I don't understand. People are basically good and I care a lot, but bad things constantly happen to me and to others. Maybe there really are some no-good S.O.B.s out there, after all. Perhaps the group doesn't have the answers. But I'm not sure if I know the questions any more."

A Level 6 thinker may begin to rediscover things within the self that are apart from friends, people, and acceptance. Self-confidence and a different kind of inner peace develop. They no longer need to be loved — they'd prefer it, but don't need it. A whole new set of questions may arise once the Level 6 needs are satiated. Life turns into a kaleidoscope of unique happenings, things to learn, and diversities to understand. The person accepts that harmony is sometimes impossible, that togetherness is not always good, and that it is possible to be autonomous without interfering with or using others. This is the transition from Level 6 to Level 7 Cognitive.

Level 7: Cognitive

The person adding Level 7 thinking to the repertoire has traversed the previous six to enable the opening up of this new type of thinking. There are lots of problems to solve before one gets to Level 7, and most of us are consumed by Level 3, 4, 5, and 6 concerns — conflict, purpose, success, and who we are. That's one reason there is still a limited amount of Level 7 thinking around and why, for most of us, it is only active in very particular aspects of our lives. Information Age technologies and living off the attainments of the previous six Levels have made the awareness of Level 7 possible.

With the shift to 7, external subsistence needs become obsolete. Physical power, rules, regulations, guidelines, approval from others, money, prestige, love, and fellowship are all fine and dandy, but none is essential to a Level 7. The Level 7 thinker appreciates the fine things in life, but requires none of them. Fear of the boss, survival, social acceptance, or even death, are of little or no concern. 7s conquer fear.

People activating Level 7 have arrived at the first of what Graves called "the being levels." Built on the foundation of Levels 1 through 6, the 7th opens the possibilities of psychological freedom. This is a state of autonomy, inner-directedness, high functionality, and cognizant complexity. It's the fourth "I"-oriented Level (the previous "I" Levels are 1, 3, and 5), taking the individual out of the community and away from its constraints, but maintaining a set of principled responsibilities.

People operating in this mode have confidence in their abilities to survive in virtually any situation. They are intrigued with existence itself and enjoy living just to observe the process of life. Although those at Level 7 don't have a driving need for a circle of friends, they can be friendly and most often have relationships. These relationships are often quite successful and frequently include those of widely differing values.

From the Level 7s perspective, nothing is universally right or wrong, good or bad. Everything is judged within its context and the person's principles — situational ethics, for example. Things are good and bad in terms of their impact on overall processes, long-range implications, and the best information available.

The success/failure dichotomy is nonsense at Level 7. With nothing to prove and evaluation internalized, failure is a learning experience which causes reconsideration but no shame. Success is based on self-perceived ranges of what was possible versus what actually happened. There will be explanation and analysis, but rarely excuses or fault-finding. Sometimes naively honest and discomfortingly straightforward, thinking at Level 7 is never ego-defensive or deceitful.

When one engages Level 7 thinking, concerns for security drop away as the desire to simply understand rises. While those centered around Level 4 suffer the guilt of original sin (or equivalent) and those focused at Level 6 feel the pain of a species struggling to find peace with itself, Level 7 thinkers are at peace with themselves. It's not fatalism or resignation to a master plan, but the view that each movement is interesting and one had best make the most of it. This sometimes leads to an appearance of childlike (not child-ish) behavior, uninhibitedness, and spontaneity.

Level 7 thinking is complex. Awareness is heightened to unusual things and aspects of events that those wrapped up in lower level concerns may overlook because of concentrated attention. For instance, after a very important conference with a bunch of very important people, you might hear a comment about "the interestingly crafted ashtray" or the "elegantly designed hinges on the conference room door." Many people would ignore these elements, criticize them, or covet them. The person at Level 7 processes a huge amount of information and just tries to appreciate it.

One day I was having lunch with a Level 7 person at the local "greasy spoon." We were sitting at the counter when suddenly, out of the blue, he leaned over and said enthusiastically, "Look at that." I looked around, couldn't see anything, and went back to my burger.

My friend was staring at the grill. I looked to where he was staring and only saw the grease-stained covering over the exhaust fan. I asked, "What are you talking about?" "That formica over the grill," he replied. "Isn't that outstanding?" All I saw was a disgusting blue panel with pink and brown streaks. To the Level 7 brain, it was a study in patterns and contrasts, wearing the stories of a million burgers and a zillion fries. The formica was a mosaic of diner-ness to my friend. To me, it was more worthy of a call to the Health Department than the Museum of Modern Art.

Someone with Level 6 thinking sees beauty in nature and things that are natural — extensions of the life force and the great chain of being. Walking through an old barn, this Level 6 person is fascinated with the exposed beams, rubs them to absorb the spirit of the place, and dreams of the stories those logs could tell. Level 7 finds meaning in formica, plastic, and plexiglass as well. In marketing to Level 6, words like "all natural," "organic" and "hand-made" are appealing. "Artificial," "man-made," and "plastic" are turn-offs to Level 6 thinking.

Level 7 thinkers often appreciate things those with less comprehensive world views do not. They may appear to be living ahead of their time, or at least to be out of sync with most everyone else. That's why we see so little Level 7 prominent in politics or even the corporate world. People living in lower systems look at Level 7s like they're nuts, odd, and strange. There's nothing in particular wrong with them — it's hard for the observers to explain — but the person is perceived as weird, anyway.

Those at Level 4 reminisce about the past; Level 5s set goals and strategize for the future; and Level 6s strive to get in touch with the here-and-now. Level 7s aren't aligned with past, present, or future; there's no need to fight the cosmos. Level 7s are interested in process.

When asked why they do things, people operating out of Level 7 say, "Because I chose to ... ," "I wanted to ... ," or "Since it was what needed to be done ..." These motivators take precedence over material gain, prestige, recognition, the need to be liked, rules, or others' expectations. One acts because one has decided to. In the process, Level 7 functioners seem to get the most out of life, milking every ounce out of events, activities, and happenings.

Abraham Maslow refers to this skill as being involved in a peak experience. Level 7 living involves a series of peak experiences throughout almost all activities. Maslow used the Japanese Zen-based word muga for this present-moment awareness. It is a state of experiencing something wholeheartedly, totally, without thinking of anything else, but just being without hesitation, inhibition, or fear of criticism. Level 7s have mastered the art of transcending time and space.

Time matters at Level 7, but not scheduled time or efficiency in time. Control of one's time is the key, whether it be to think, play, work, create, meditate, make love; and that control will not be surrendered to outside forces. The Level 7 person is not driven by the clock or imposed schedules. Response to schedules is a matter of choice, not compulsion.

Have you ever become so involved and interested in something that you almost lose track of what else is going on? That's somewhat like Level 7 thinking, except that the person doesn't lose touch. One is highly focused and generally aware at the same time.

Level 4s question, if there is life after death. Level 7s determine *where there is life after birth*. And they proceed to experience it to supernatural heights.

As you can imagine, Level 7s are difficult to manage; they think the sun doesn't rise until they open their eyes. Graves states:

"... He will not follow a standard operating procedure. He will produce well — but only when the manager-producer role is reversed.

"... He rebels against the idea that it is management's prerogative to plan or organize work methods without consulting help, ... management insists that he conform ... he refuses."

Since Level 7s have much to contribute but refuse to be told how to do things, the appropriate management style is to achieve agreement on objectives with the 7 and then fully support the 7. This facilitative style of management unleashes the 7's productivity, thus enhancing the attainment of the organization's objectives. Level 7s are dangerous managers. Their intense desire to enjoy living and excitement encourages 7s to view chaotic and hellish actions as intriguing and extremely enjoyable as long as they are purposeful. A smooth-running, orderly and purposeful operation is boring to any Level 7. Can you imagine a Level 7 manager, standing off and observing the employees as if in an experimental box; and, when things begin to run smoothly and efficiently, the Level 7 manager merely shakes the box a little to stir things up? Level 7s believe you cannot have any type of growth without dissonance. People cannot grow physically, psychologically, emotionally, if they are comfortable.

So, a Level 7 person is experiencing life to its fullest, having a ball with all of life's inconsistencies, chaos, confusion, nonsensical happenings. A Level 7 person is appreciating peak experiences daily. An individual has seemingly no limits, is free, is experiencing heaven on earth. All of a sudden, one morning, the Level 7 wakes up and decides: This isn't what life is all about; concludes: I don't have all the answers and realizes: There is something bigger than life itself. At this point, some Level 7s begin to grow into 8s.

CHAPTER TWELVE

UNDERSTANDING THE MENTAL STAIRCASE

The Level 8 is referred to as experientialistic. In essence, what happens is 7th Level individuals, after experiencing life to its fullest, with all of life's inconsistencies, chaos, and confusion, begin to grow into 8s as they accept existential dichotomies. Level 8s value wonder, awe, reverence, humility, fusion, integration, simplicity, and unity.

Level 8s communicate with an external force, usually via meditation or intuition. This relationship with the outside force resembles a partnership rather than a superior-subordinate relationship; it is a oneness with the universe. The life and work of Walter Russell, as reported by Glenn Clark, provide many illustrations of Level 8 thinking. For example, Russell stated:

> No greater proof than my experience is needed to prove to the doubting world that all knowledge exists in the mind universe of light — which is God — that all mind is one mind, that men do not have separate minds, and that all knowledge can be obtained from the universal source of all-knowledge by becoming one with the source.

Many great thinkers of all ages have believed in a unit consciousness. They have believed that an individual's "stored information" is not limited to their own memories of past experiences or learned facts. "There is one mind common to all individual man," said Emerson, who, according to Maxwell Maltz, compared our individual minds to the inlets in an ocean of universal mind. Edison believed he got some of his ideas from a source outside of himself.

This oneness is sometimes referred to as *the secret of the universe.* Each individual is an integral part of this oneness and all knowledge stems from this oneness. All a person needs to do to become all-knowing is to tap the eternal truth of the universal source, which is done by turning inside via meditation rather than looking outside for the answer.

To illustrate, a Level 8 displays a painting and asks the average person, "Is this painting real?"

The obvious reply is "Yes."

The 8 continues, "How do you know it is real?"

The average person responds, "Because I can see it, I can touch it, I can appreciate it, if necessary, I can destroy it."

The 8 counters, "No, that's not what makes it real; what makes it real is the thought process that went into making it. If there were no thought process, there would be no painting. The canvas, the paint, the frame are insignificant. The only things in life that are real are thought processes. The same is true with the universe. The only real parts of the universe are those thought processes that make up the universe. For instance, as the force constructed the universe, it was similar to the artist who developed this painting. The artist put thinking and feeling into the painting; in other words, put part of oneself into it and that idea, that self, cannot be snuffed out by physically destroying the painting. The force constructed the universe out of self; that is, everything, everyone, every anything is inter-connected. We are all joined by invisible strands called cosmos; we are all one."

What difference does it make whether we are all one or not? To a Level 8 it makes a great deal of difference. For instance, the average person knows that the thumb is a part of one's body; therefore, it would make no sense to hit the thumb with a hammer. To a Level 8, we are all one; therefore, it makes no sense to hurt our fellow man because when we hurt our fellow man, we hurt ourselves.

Level 8s not only believe in oneness, they live as if a oneness exists.

Walter Russell, when he was 15 years old, was asked by his girl-friend if he would take her to the opera. He agreed, but she quickly brought it to his attention that she was referring to the entire series while he was thinking of one performance. The series would cost him $79.60 and since he was earning only $12 a week, he exclaimed, "That is impossible!"

She looked at him in amazement, "I don't believe it."

"You don't believe what, that I don't have the money?" Walter replied.

She retorted, "No, I don't believe you said it was impossible. I've never heard you say something was impossible."

Walter thought for a moment and replied, "That's it, we're going to the opera."

When it came time to get advanced tickets, Walter found himself waiting in a long line with only $6 in his pocket. The average person would think Walter Russell had gone Looney Tunes, but that is what we like about **PeopleWise**®. If you can get inside someone's head and think like they think, you can understand their behavior because people think rationally. You see, Walter only had $6 in his pocket, but he had the secret of the universe in his head; and he knew he would have the $79.60 by the time he got to the head of the line.

As the line began to slowly move, unexpectedly, Walter was approached by a man who asked, "Would you like to sell your place in line for $5?" An ordinary person would take the $5, run to the back of the line, and hope someone would buy his place in line again, again, again ... Not Walter. He quickly pulled from his pocket a small notebook and a pencil and asked, "Would you like to have the tickets delivered to your door?"

The man gave Walter the money for the tickets plus $5 and Walter wrote down the customer's name and address. Holding the money between his fingers like a bookmaker, he became a magnet drawing scores of people to him, and, according to Glenn Clark, by the time Walter Russell reached the box office, he had the amount necessary for the entire series plus an additional $110.

But that isn't the amazing part of this true story. The amazing thing is, *not one person asked Walter's name nor asked for a receipt.* You see, when you are in touch with the cosmos, when you are a Level 8, when you are at one with the world, people trust you, people believe you; Level 8s give off vibrations of truth, honesty, and sincerity. Asking for a receipt from Walter Russell would be no different than asking for a receipt from Mahatma Gandhi or Mother Teresa. It is unthinkable.

You guessed it; a person goes along meditating, communicating with the universe, developing a sensitivity for oneness and all of a sudden, one day, realizes there is something more to life, something bigger than the universe itself, and they begin to grow into 9s. I am going to stop here for a minute, because there aren't enough 9s in the world today to even make it worth our time to talk about them but, more important, you wouldn't believe it any way. What I am going to do is share with you some of the intricacies of this mental staircase and some of its inter-workings.

To begin with, most people do not fit neatly into any single Level. Most people are a combination of Levels and, as you read and study the Levels, you probably could identify with characteristics from each Level. Most people can identify with bits and pieces of each Level because they have open personalities. Open personalities are a blend of several Levels.

Figure 12-1 illustrates an open Level 5. In this example, 50 percent to 60 percent of the person's thinking, acting, and behaving is based in Level 5. The person also has some Level 4 and some 6, and a little 3 and 7.

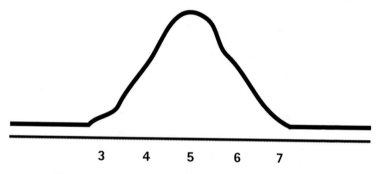

| 3 | 4 | 5 | 6 | 7 |

Figure 12-1. Open personality type at 5th Level

A few people have closed personalities, as illustrated in Figure 12-2. Here we have a closed Level 5 where 90 percent to 95 percent of the person's thinking, acting, and behaving is based in Level 5. People with closed personalities have trouble relating to, understanding, or accepting individuals that are functioning on Levels different than their own Level. Individuals with closed personalities have a low tolerance for differences, while open personality individuals have a high tolerance for differences.

For individuals who are interested in improving their psychological and emotional development, two types of growth are possible. One type of growth broadens a person's perspectives within a Level; that is, a person grows from a closed personality to an open personality. Persons with open personalities are more flexible, have a greater tolerance for differences in other people, can draw from a larger repertoire of ideas, concepts, and skills when confronted with a problem and, in general, have a larger, healthier psychological base from which to work. Growing from a closed personality to an open personality is referred to as intrasystemic growth. *Intra* means within or inward, *system* refers to the psychological Levels; thus, intrasystemic growth implies growth within a Level.

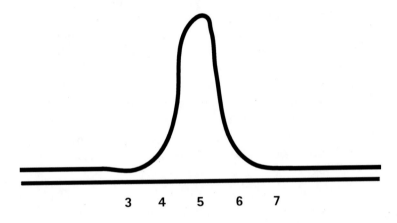

Figure 12-2. Closed personality type at 5th Level

Another type of growth would involve movement up the psychological staircase, that is, moving from a 3 to a 4, or a 4 to a 5, or a 5 to a 6, etc. This type of growth is referred to as intersystemic growth. Inter means between or among, system still refers to the psychological Levels; thus, intersystemic growth implies growth between or among the Levels.

The conditions for both intrasystemic and intersystemic growth are similar. They are:
1. The needs at the present Level must be met and satisfied.
2. Dissonance or a challenge must present itself.
3. The individual must be exposed to different types of thinking, acting, and/or behaving. This may come in the form of an insight or an awareness.

Meeting the needs of the present Level refers to satisfying an individual's basic needs to the point of relative contentment. The needs focused on at each of the Levels are:

Level One, Reactive: Physiological
Level Two, Tribalistic: Safety and Assurance
Level Three, Egocentric: Survival and Power
Level Four, Absolutist: Security
Level Five, Materialist: Prestige and Material Things
Level Six, Sociocentric: Friendship and Affiliation
Level Seven, Cognitive: Existence and Freedom to Live
Level Eight, Experientialistic: Experience and Mind Exploration

As mentioned earlier, the concept of meeting people's needs and accepting them for what they are appeals to me. I do not mean to imply that people will not or cannot (behaviorally) change without their individual psychological needs being met first. However, I suggest that if the needs are not met in a (behaviorally) changed person, the minute the pressure is off or the minute the reinforcers are removed, the individual will more than likely revert to the previous psychological Level. To me, this is so important that it cannot be overemphasized. For instance, before an individual can *effectively and consistently* motivate, persuade, sell, counsel, teach, or manage another person, the motivator, persuader, salesperson, counselor, teacher, or manager must first gain the trust of the prospect, must first establish rapport, must first meet needs. But one of the real attributes of **PeopleWise® Motivation** is that it gives us a plan and tells us how to meet those many and varied needs of specific individuals.

The presence of dissonance or the insertion of a challenge means nothing more than that the potentially changing individual is uncomfortable. No one grows or wants to grow if they are contented, complacent or comfortable. Here I am referring to being psychologically uncomfortable, that is, confused, puzzled, worried. As an individual becomes uncomfortable, the natural reaction is to seek comfort; if the person is confused, puzzled or worried, the person seeks answers. Dissonance and/or challenge set the stage for growth.

Being exposed to different types of thinking, acting, and/or behaving refers to exposure to other Levels of thinking. For instance, for intrasystemic growth the individual is exposed to the two adjacent Levels and for intersystemic growth the individual is exposed to the next succeeding Level.

Let's say an individual is a closed Level 5 and we want to open the person up. First, we meet as many Level 5 needs as we can. We assist them in getting promoted, we encourage them to buy things, we brag on their car, clothes, the way they look, smell, and act. We gain the Level 5's confidence and trust and, just as Level 5 thinks he or she knows all the answers, thinks they are succeeding, thinks they are important, we insert dissonance. We can insert dissonance in a variety of ways. One easy way would be to openly question Level 5's motives or abilities. All we want to do is throw the Level 5 off just enough to make them uncomfortable. We would never advocate a divorce, but if you have ever experienced a divorce or if you have ever been close to someone in the midst of one, then you know what dissonance is. People experiencing dissonance get confused, question themselves, and seek answers. During dissonance the mind gets active — *very active*. As the Level 5 seeks answers, we expose the person to both Level 4 and 6th Level thinking, acting, and behaving. We do this through readings, movies, new acquaintances, etc. In essence, we psychologically pull the 5 open. Notice, we would not accomplish anything if we inserted dissonance in an individual whose needs had not been met. Inserting dissonance in individuals who are not confident, not satisfied, not contented, leads to super confusion, hypertension, and chaos; and, all in all, is not psychologically healthy.

By the way, if the 5 were open and the goal was intersystemic growth, the exposure would center exclusively around Level 6 thinking, acting, and behaving. Growth is a touchy business and we don't recommend playing mind games with people; but understanding the growth process allows us to understand the behavior of others as well as our own behavior, and allows us to predict subsequent behavior beyond chance. For instance, if dissonance gets too great and it develops into trauma, individuals drop two levels and subsequently grow until they hit their heads on the next succeeding psychological Level. As an example of dropping levels under stress, one could make an educated guess that Nancy Reagan (a Level 4-5) turned to astrology (Level 2 behavior) after the President was shot. Let's take another example. Nixon would have been considered a closed 5. He was political, calculative, goal-oriented, high on drive, etc. Then the Watergate trauma set in. As trauma set in, he dropped to a Level 3 — remember, he physically struck his press secretary — then he moves to a 4 — remember him excessively quoting from the Bible — then he moves back to 5 — and then briefly to a 6 — remember, he publicly denounced the Alaskan pipeline, which previously he fervently supported.

When dealing in human behavior, you are never dealing in absolutes, but you are always confronted with probabilities — how probable is it that A will happen in B situation. No one would ever have believed you if you had predicted that the President of the United States — a statesman, an attorney, a proud person — would actually physically strike another person. Yet, after it happened, people would have thought you were psychic when, in fact, you had only mastered an understanding of **PeopleWise®** Motivation. Thus, as with any good theory, you were able to predict human behavior beyond chance.

Let's take a **PeopleWise®** guess at the first Spinks-Ali fight. When Muhammad Ali was Cassius Clay, he performed as a 3 or 3-4 combination. When he changed his name to Muhammad Ali he was telling us, "I'm a 4." As we know, he accumulated wealth and grew to 5 and, as he became benevolent and charitable, he began to hit his head on 6. Spinks was a 3-4. We conclude this because he reportedly drank beer and ate raw eggs for breakfast. Several days prior to the fight, Ali, for the first time, got in a skirmish with his religious advisors and ordered them out of the training camp. This behavior would indicate that he was moving toward a 5-6 combination and moving away from 4. So we had a 3 (Spinks) in the ring with a 5-6 (Ali). Anyone who knows anything about the theory behind **PeopleWise®** Motivation and anyone who likes to bet would have put money on Spinks, but, better yet, Ali was giving fifteen-to-one odds. Fifteen-to-one odds on a 3 fighting a 5-6 wasn't even a gamble; it was an *investment.* Now look what happened: Spinks wins, subsequently grows into a 4-5, mostly 5; Ali experiences dissonance, subsequently gets religion and begins to train like a 3-4. Now we have a rematch of a 3-4 (Ali) pitted against a 5 (Spinks). Once again, it's like going to the bank. Remember, a theory makes sense out of chaos, allows you to predict beyond chance, and then provides you with a plan for selecting significant variables that, when altered, result in changes and outcomes; that is, they allow us to cause things to happen. Now that you are beginning to understand the theory behind **PeopleWise® Motivation**, do you see how we could psychologically help Ali make a comeback; do you see how you could motivate him to train like a 3, think like a 3, fight like a 3? Now we understand why "Eye of the Tiger" in Rocky III rose to number one; it was real, at least we thought it was real. Knowing the theory behind **PeopleWise® Motivation** gives us an insight or at least a little understanding of how and why Tyson bit off Holyfield's ear, Saddam Hussein stayed in power so long, Bill Clinton said, "I did not have sex with that woman," and so on.

Learning more about the theory behind **PeopleWise® Motivation** gets fun, doesn't it? About this time I really get excited because from here on we begin to understand that the theory is not a categorizing plan to place people in Levels. As mentioned in the beginning, it really is a staircase with identifiable landings. It is a scheme for understanding how to motivate ourselves as well as others.

Now let's take another look at the theory (see Figure 12-3). Here we see similarities between odd and even numbered Levels. Even numbered Levels tend to be reflective, introvertive, reactive, that's the "we"; while odd numbered Levels tend to be projective, extrovertive, active, and proactive, that's the "I." One would think that an individual would psychologically grow toward a compatible type of thinking, acting, and behaving, but apparently, most people psychologically swing from opposite Level to opposite Level, as a pendulum swings back and forth. Conceptually, normal growth goes something like this: persons are born as closed 1s; as the physiological needs are met, they open up to such a degree that they hook onto Level 2. After hooking onto Level 2, they close up a little to get a better grasp on who and what they are; then, as their safety needs are met, they open up to such a degree that they hook onto Level 3. After hooking onto Level 3, they close up a little, then open up and hook onto 4, etc.

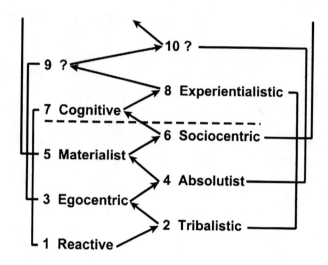

Figure 12-3. PeopleWise® Motivation Staircase

Notice the line separating 6s and 7s. This line represents a rebirth; some have referred to it as: the individual at Level 7 is psychologically reborn — for the first time, this person cannot be motivated through external events, actions, or things. This person is truly a psychological thinking being. Moving from a Level 6 to a 7 is the most difficult type of growth between any of the other Levels because the 6 must conquer fear before moving to 7. Most, if not all, 7s have rubbed elbows with death or have witnessed death at first hand.

What the lines on the sides of the staircase are depicting is: a Level 7 is a recycled 1, a Level 8 is a recycled 2; a Level 9 is a recycled 3, etc. Now we have a theory about psychological development that has no limits; that is, humankind's ability to develop psychologically is infinite. Furthermore, we are able to have some insight into what constitutes high level development.

Think about 2s and 8s. Both Levels are somewhat mystical, both have a belief about an external Force, both individuals would be considered a little unique, if not weird, by western culture standards. To 8s, the "tribe" is the planet. What primarily separates the 2 from the 8 is the concept of death and control. Level 2s have not conquered the fear of death and they are purely reactive to the environment, believing they have little or no control over it. Eights have no fear of anything and believe they are All-Knowing and can control anything and everything. Crudely put, 2s are subservient to the superstition, while 8s make the superstition work for them.

Now think about 3s and 9s. Threes settled the American West. Nines will take us to other planets. Threes are physically power-oriented, but they are indiscriminate with the power; that is, they fight anyone and anything to survive. Level 9s will exhibit physical power but it will be discriminating and supposedly for the betterment of society. As an example, Level 9s would advocate mercy killing of individuals in the back wards of institutions, euthanasia, and abortion. How could Level 9s advocate killing without letting it bother their consciences? Keep in mind, persons 7 and above have not only conquered the fear of death, they don't even believe it exists — they believe in an unfolding and refolding process. Thus, they have no qualms about advocating taking the life of a "vegetable" in the back ward of the institution because they don't believe they are killing the person, they are actually assisting the person in the unfolding and refolding process. So the next time you read in the paper about someone suggesting a patient being removed from a life support system, don't think they are crazy or mentally deranged. There is a strong likelihood that the person is involved in some Level 9 thinking where *quality* of life takes on a different meaning than *quantity* of life. Knowing the theory behind **PeopleWise® Motivation** possibly gives us insights into the thoughts and thinking of Jack Kevorkian. Might Dr. Kevorkian have some 9ish thinking in him?

Quickly, let's look at 4s and 10s. Level 4s believe in a supreme being and view death as real. Level 10s think of themselves as part of the supreme being and can't even conceive of the concept of death. In other words, 10s think they are God or think they are disciples of God.

Don't let **PeopleWise® Motivation** disturb or scare you. It is just a theory based on how I believe people think. It is not the truth, but it does provide a means that helps us make sense out of chaos; lets us predict things beyond chance; and provides us with some ideas on how we can help ourselves and others grow, mature, and develop. We can use the **PeopleWise® Motivation** staircase for real.

CHAPTER THIRTEEN

USING THE STAIRCASE FOR REAL

Wall-covering company asked me to analyze individuals who shopped for wallpaper. I discovered that Level 4s, 5s, and 6s seemed to be evenly divided among our sample and, although specific types of paper seemed to appeal to each of the types of buyers, I noticed all the selling techniques to be very similar. All of the selling centered around a counseling format. The salesperson determined what room(s) were to be covered and a little about what the customer preferred in terms of pattern, color, and texture. Then the sales approach was to display books upon books containing samples of various types of wallpaper. Seldom, if ever, did the customer buy on the first visit. After discovering this, I decided to have the salespersons complete an instrument that would determine *their* Level of preference. As I suspected, I found that over 90 percent of the salespersons scored as Level 6s.

I waited outside in my car until just the right customer arrived. It was a little past noon when a deep green BMW drove up and parked next to the door in a no-parking spot (fire zone). A well-dressed woman in a pin-striped business suit and alligator heels rushed in. Ten minutes later she came out, empty handed, and drove away. I followed. She went to a mall up the street and ran into another wallpaper store. Again she came out. Again I followed. She went to another store and, as before, came out empty-handed. As I continued to follow, she proceeded, apparently back to work. Three stores in one hour.

Two weeks later I phoned her. This was accomplished because she had left her business card with our salesperson. I mentioned to her that it had been brought to my attention that she had visited our store. I was curious as to whether she had purchased any paper and how she had found our selections. She indicated that she had purchased some wallpaper (from another store), although she had found our store friendly, pleasant, and containing an excellent selection. Then I asked the key question, "How might we improve our service?"

She came back with, "Get better at getting to what the customer wants in fewer questions. Present a few of the best options to select from and streamline the purchasing process. You also might want to investigate some type of computer selection process. But keep it simple," she continued.

I asked, "How few should the options be?"

She retorted, "Six to eight."

You guessed it; she was a Level 5 and we were trying to sell her as if she were a Level 6. In fact, we were trying to sell everyone as if they were 6s.

To increase the skills of the sales staff and to increase the options for dealing with different types of customers, we developed a selling program based on **PeopleWise®** methods and began to sell brain-to-brain.

PeopleWise® Motivation techniques, when applied to sales, result in increased volume and profits, plus delighted customers. After reviewing more than 100 PeopleWise® Profile Instruments filled out by customers visiting a Volkswagen dealership in Florida, I discovered over 70 percent were identified as Level 6, sociocentrics. While researching buyers at a Buick dealership in Georgia, I found that over 80 percent of the individuals considering luxury vehicles were Level 5s, materialists, while over 60 percent of those considering economy cars could be identified as Level 4s, absolutists.

Individuals seem to have a tendency to shop for automobiles that match their personalities and, furthermore, they seem to appreciate a sales approach that is in concert with how they wish to be handled.

It all began one sunny afternoon in 1984 at the Critz Used Car Lot in Savannah, Georgia. I was standing with the other salespersons in the showroom, looking out onto the lot when all of a sudden, a 25ish, long-haired, ear-ringed, individual drove up on a motorcycle. Before I could move, all the other salespeople disappeared — some went to their offices, some to the restroom, and one out back for a smoke.

The motorcyclist parked his two-wheeler and walked around a Volkswagen van. Being a non-smoker, not having to go to the restroom, and not liking to be confined to my office, I wandered out to introduce myself.

As I walked out, I noticed white lettering across the back of his navy blue tee shirt, "Save the whales." An old beat-up bumper sticker was stuck to the left saddlebag which read, "Split wood not atoms"; it was just below the peace sign.

His name was Bruce; he liked to camp and was a skilled canoeist. His eyes were blue, his hair hung just below his shoulders, he was wearing docksiders with no socks, and he had a leather friendship bracelet around his left ankle. Yes, no question about it — I had my hands on a real, whale-saving, one-worlder, you-are-the-children, antinuker, Level 6, if I ever saw one.

I didn't know much about selling, but I did know you can't sell a 6. Instead, you let a 6 buy. I also knew 6s don't purchase anything on their first visit. They reflect, think, and shop. Sixes must like and trust the person they deal with. They hate authority figures and they are very consumer literate, i.e., they research the products before buying.

I asked a series of questions and, with my best body language and eye contact, I absorbed everything he said. I found out that he was interested in a truck to use for all his friends to put their gear in while they traveled across the country. He had read *Consumer Guide* and *Consumer Reports* and knew exactly what he wanted, except for the size of the cargo space.

We went to a truck he had his eye on. This was an interesting truck because it had been on the lot for over a year, was new — not used, but the cargo portion extended over the cab and was a little unusual. Bruce liked the cargo area. He figured he could put a mattress in the cargo part above the cab and use it as a sleeping area. He said he had never seen a cargo area like this and the more he talked, the more I liked it. He knew everything about this truck. He even got under the truck to show me some aspects of the muffler. I'd never been under a truck before.

Although I was tempted to sell him, I knew better, so when he exhausted himself telling me everything he knew about the truck, I asked him if he had been over to the Ford dealership. He said, "no," so I suggested he might check them out. He shook my hand, mounted up, and drove off.

When I walked back into the showroom, the other salespeople snickered and avoided me as if I had the plague. The next day Bruce returned. I was in the back room at the time, so one of the other salespersons opened the door and explained, "The wild one's back." As Bruce and I went to my office, he talked about a trip he was planning. We got out an atlas and charted the trip to New Mexico. We never talked much about the truck, but before leaving, he indicated that Ford didn't have anything he wanted and asked if I had any other suggestions. I told him trucks were a little out of my field, but I noticed some trucks on an independent used car lot about a quarter of a mile up the road. He left.

Two days later Bruce returned to buy the truck with the unique cargo space. Here was a pure 6, using a 6 technique. More importantly, two months later he referred a Level 6 friend who ended up buying a Volkswagen van. When **PeopleWise®** methods are appropriately applied, average salespersons can substantially increase their repertoire of skills as they master brain-to-brain selling.

I first discovered that knowledge of **PeopleWise® Motivation** could be used in betting on various sporting events, especially those that were aggressive and violent (such as football and boxing). By subscribing to various football magazines and studying what was written about various coaches and significant players, I could assign a level to most teams. Significant players were identified as linebackers on defense, and on offense, the ends, quarterbacks, and any famous or highly paid player. For example, when Joe Namath played with the New York Jets, they played like Level 6s. The Washington Redskins, under George Allen, were coached like 4s; the Dallas Cowboys, under Tom Landry, were a 4-5 combination; while the Pittsburgh Steelers practiced and played like closed 5s; and the St. Louis Cardinals were at the time Level 6s.

During the first four games of each season, Level 4 teams tend to beat the point spread over Level 5 teams. In other words, no matter who was favored to win, during the first four season games, Level 4 teams were by far the best bet. This makes sense when you think about it. Level 4 players practice, even without a contract. If there is a player strike, it is not unusual for Level 4 players to practice even without their coach, whereas Level 5s have a tendency to wait at home and remain off the field until the strike has been settled. Level 6s don't take practicing seriously before, during, or after the season. Practice to Level 6s should be fun. They make practice fun.

During the last five to seven games of the season, Level 5 teams tend to beat the point spread when pitted against 4s. By that time the 5s get together and say, "If we are going to make it to the Super Bowl, we'd better get our act together." During the latter part of the season, Level 4 teams seem to be plagued with more than their share of injuries. They seem to believe the only way to win is to keep hitting again and again and again and again; they are not too imaginative and they are far from creative. They keep going back to basics. They actually believe it is their duty to play hurt. In fact, it is honorable to play hurt.

Level 6 teams are wild and creative. On any given day they can beat any given team, but they win through surprise, razzle-dazzle, and just plain luck. Never bet on a Level 6 team or, for that matter, never bet against them. As far as the point spread is concerned, they are inconsistent; the computer can't keep track of the 6's style of play. As a standard practice, I never bet on any Level 6 teams, but I love to watch them play.

As I collected information on teams, I found I could not assign a level to every team. Several teams were identified as "no-number teams." These teams didn't seem to have anything or anybody pulling them together in a cohesive direction, purpose, or philosophy. A "no-number team" appeared to think they could win if they learned the plays, practiced the fundamentals, and executed well. Level 4 teams believe you win through blood, sweat, and sacrifice; Level 5 teams believe you win by calculating and out-thinking your opponent, as if in a giant chess game. Level 6 teams believe the element of surprise has won many a battle.

An interesting observation was that when certain Level 4 and 5 teams played "no number teams," they would *consistently* either beat the point spread or not beat the point spread. For instance, I found that when the Dallas Cowboys (Level 4-5 combination) played a "no number team," they seldom beat the point spread, whereas the Pittsburgh Steelers (5s) almost always beat the point spread when they were pitted against a "no number team."

So during the first four games of the season I bet 4s over 5s, never bet on 6s, and I kept track of how 4s and 5s showed against no numbers. During the middle of the season, when 4s and 5s were either getting hurt or trying to make up their minds if it was worth it all, I placed bets on 4s and 5s that played "no number teams" based upon the data I had kept earlier. The latter part of the season I went with the 5s. Over three seasons the strategy held: I never failed to predict the majority of the outcomes. One season I topped 80 percent.

After three years of successfully applying **PeopleWise® Motivation** to betting, I was given an opportunity to advise an NFL team. I was first invited to present at a general meeting to the head coach and assistant coaches. After a five-hour meeting, I was invited to return to develop a strategy for implementing **PeopleWise® Motivation** techniques in the game of football.

I began interviewing various players to develop **PeopleWise®** personal profiles on each player. An individual personal profile was developed to determine the current level of functioning and some of the primary motivational keys. The following are actual examples of some abbreviated **PeopleWise®** personal profiles. Letters have been substituted for actual names for purposes of confidentiality.

Player A
Level 4 (open)
rules & schedules are motivators
high expectations
time is motivating

This player should be no problem to motivate or manage in the present system. I would suggest he be taught how to keep his own training (daily) records and I would have an assistant coach go over the records with him about once or twice a month. Prayer is important to him and a prayer group (with you joining in occasionally) might be motivating.

Player B
7 or open 5
intelligent and family oriented
variety, surprise

This player will function under any system, but to highly motivate him he needs to be exposed to variety, novelty, and surprise. He rolls with the punches and knows his own limitations. He feels 95 percent of his playing is mental. He has resolved a lot of problems other players are experiencing and he could be used as a discussion leader or just a friend to share his ideas and thinking. This player is presently doing a lot of introspection, yet he is psychologically one of the most healthy individuals I talked to. The question is not how to manage and motivate Player B, but how to use him and his skills to motivate others.

Player C
2-3 combination
sensitive – jokester

This player is learning disabled yet he probably learns average to above average from imitation and immediate visual feedback. He could benefit from being trained via a video tape unit. The visual feedback must be immediate. Player C gets lost in words, and the worst way to teach or motivate him is through words. I would say you should put him beside someone who is emotional and he will follow suit. Player C could benefit from a counselor, just someone to occasionally listen to him. He likes to talk. He has a need to talk. However, often his talk distracts others.

Player E
Level 5
pseudo intellectual
lazy
time is important – possible motivator
rewards and bonuses are motivators
(sometimes can't get up for game; this indicates lack of intensity)

This player came to the session and explained that he was busy and could only talk for about 10 minutes. He then asked how much of the conversation was confidential. I explained none. He said OK and proceeded to tell me a lot of personal things about himself and fellow players. I occasionally reminded him the session was not confidential. I don't believe he really cared whether it was or it wasn't.

I would recommend that he be placed on a written psychological contract indicating what he wants, what the team wants, and what the team can actually provide. This player seems to psychologically have potential -- through negotiation of a psychological contract he could be motivated to (1) come to camp on weight and (2) train and stay in shape. He should be objectively evaluated at regular intervals (at least once a week). Please note, poor management will result in this player never getting into physical shape. This player will emotionally wear you down if you continue to apply your present motivation and management strategies with him.

The following is a specific example of how **PeopleWise® Motivation** was used to assist a player in improving his performance: We focused on a particular player that had trouble psyching himself up. Later, it became apparent he had an open personality but was developing into a 6. Level 6s don't have any business in football, especially in power positions. This particular player verbalized how difficult it was to psyche himself up, and how he actually felt uneasy when someone got hurt, even if it was the opposition. We improved this particular player's performance by never mentioning the opposing players by name. The less he knew about the opposing player's life, family, etc., the better he played. Let it be understood that football teams have access to some very detailed reports regarding the opposition; sometimes this information is personal. We prepared this player to look at the opposition as machines with predictable responses. Next, we encouraged this player to decide on particular defensive strategies for each game. We taught this player the basics of psychocybernetics and meditation, similar to what was presented in Chapters 1-5. Psychocybernetics taught him to mentally rehearse what was to happen before it happened. Later we found that through psychocybernetics he could mentally convince himself he was not human. In other words, he developed a skill of turning himself off and on humanistically. We found he was playing with more intensity, but he lacked quickness and agility. We showed him films and timed his reactions which made him come up with the idea of thinking of himself as a panther. He cut out pictures of panthers and looked at them as he meditated. His reaction time improved over night. When this player learned what motivated him, he was psychologically in perfect control of himself on and off the field. What was most impressive was how this player learned to use his brain and emotions to handle conflicting situations. He was a quiet, sensitive, soft, warm, and loving individual employed to hit and be violent. He learned how and when to do both extremely well. He mastered mind control.

I have also discovered that **PeopleWise® Motivation** works in the legal arena as well as sports. Have you ever received a speeding ticket but didn't think you deserved it? Regardless of how you felt, did you pay the fine anyway because you felt you couldn't beat it in court?

Have you ever felt threatened to do something because if you didn't, you would be sued?

Well, you are not alone. Most people don't want to go to court; don't like to get involved in law suits; and are afraid of judges, juries, attorneys, and the entire trial process. Most people conclude that it's just not worth it; you can't fight city hall; I don't have time to get involved; thus, they avoid courtroom encounters. Yet, despite all these fears and concerns, you stand better than a 50/50 chance of going to court in some capacity.

Better than 6 percent of the general population will perform jury duty during their life time. Approximately 25 percent of the general population will be a party to some type of litigation, and almost as many will serve as witnesses in some capacity.

Most people find the practice of law scary because they have not taken the time to study the litigation process and the psychology of the courtroom. Before getting involved in various cases, I had the naive notion that the law was the law — if you violated the law and you got caught, bad things happened to you. Black is black and white is white; you were either innocent or guilty. The most important lesson I learned was that judges and juries don't make the law; *they interpret the law.* They are empowered to determine if the law was broken or not and the result is justice.

Next, I learned that judges and juries are made up of people — people who are human, people who have feelings, people who have strengths and weaknesses, people who can be reasoned with, sold, persuaded, conned, tricked ... I am not advocating that anyone con, trick, or maliciously manipulate another person, but I do want to make it perfectly clear that innocent people, or people who have extenuating circumstances, should stand up for their rights and state their case honestly, sincerely, and clearly. Furthermore, accused people must present their case in a manner that is favorable to their position and not naively in a manner that can be torn down, attacked, defeated, ridiculed, massacred, or mutilated by someone trained in the art of debate, rebuttal, and intimidation. *Justice is not the law; justice is what a judge or jury determines it is. Justice is the decision that stems from the courtroom.* The following case illustrates how to apply **PeopleWise® Motivation** to a moving vehicle violation.

You are driving down the highway when a car pulls out in front of you from a roadside service station. To avoid hitting the car, you instinctively jerk your car over to the lefthand passing lane and immediately approach a stopped car turning left. You slam on your brakes but slide into the turning vehicle. The car pulling from the service station speeds away. A patrolman comes; you explain the situation; and you get the station attendant to verify that a car pulled out. The attendant says yes, a car pulled out, but you were going too fast to stop. You are given a ticket for reckless driving even though you weren't going over the speed limit, you weren't swerving in and out of traffic, you didn't run a light, and you weren't on mind-altering drugs; in fact, you didn't do anything but hit another car. You get upset, you get mad, no — you get downright ticked; and you want to choke that little sawed-off runt of a service attendant. But chances are you won't fight it in court because it costs too much or because you don't have time. Instead, you will plead guilty.

Before pleading guilty, you must realize that judges are human. In your opinion, you were not driving recklessly and, therefore, at least give it your best shot. Judges are neither all-knowing nor omnipotent, and I have found most judges understanding and compassionate. Furthermore, traffic court judges are relatively free wheeling in their decision making. Later, I will show you how I won this actual, real case.

As early as the 16th century, Montaigne indicated that a judge's mood and humor varied from day to day and were often reflected in their decisions. Oliver Wendell Holmes, in the late 1800s, stated: "A decision is the unconscious result of instinctive prejudices and inarticulate connections," and "even the prejudices which judges share with their fellow men have a good deal more to do than the syllogism in determining the rules by which men should be governed." *In other words, judges are human, too.*

Just as judges are human, juries are composed of sensitive, feeling beings; but more importantly, members of the jury are not trained in law, and we can thank God for that. Keep in mind that just because a jury is sworn in, it is unlikely that jurors will become judicious, level-headed, rational, insightful, evaluators of the evidence presented in the courtroom. Decisions of jurors are likely to involve perceptions of people, self-concept, and the expectations of people as to age, gender, race, and physical and emotional characteristics. A jury is involved in group process and is composed of leaders and followers. Psychologists have found juries to be a Disney World in which the analysis of human behavior is exciting, alive and electric.

Attorneys have been trained in the psychology of influencing and persuading jurors. Human beings, in general, are impressionistic; and courtroom drama provides an arena to move, persuade, and alter people's thinking. No wonder there have been so many courtroom dramas on each television network since the inception of television. Brodsky captures this excitement in describing the cross-examination process of a witness as similar to Wonder Woman's being attacked by enemies firing bullets, so she moves her wrists with lightning speed. Wonder Woman's bracelets deflect each of the bullets so that they zing back at the assailant or harmlessly fall to the ground. Individuals on a witness stand find themselves in a similar position, under attack.

The witness can count on receiving a number of hostile missiles; most witnesses, however, were not bred on Paradise Island or blessed by Athena, and are not able to fend off attorneys' bullets with the speed and grace of a Wonder Woman. All too many witnesses find themselves distressed by the unfamiliar field of battle, opposed by the courtroom equivalent of super-heroes and heroines (in attorneys and other witnesses alike), and sufficiently wounded that they vow to never risk such hazards again.

Attorneys prefer psychologically attractive witnesses — married, good job, no police record, and serious demeanor. The purpose is to make a favorable impression on the jury — dressed well, but not overly dressed; tending to project credibility. Squirming, looking out the window, blushing, appearing nervous, and other nonverbal behaviors may affect a judge or juror in some way. Character witnesses are used to testify to the impeccability of the defendant's reputation, while expert witnesses are hired because they have special knowledge of some aspect of the case. Expert witnesses will present their experience, education, and other qualifications, including honors achieved, publications, and other evidence indicating authoritativeness. An attempt is made to strike a happy medium between arrogance and humility. It is of paramount importance to remember that the *cross-examination of any witness attempts to demonstrate bias or raise doubts about the accuracy of the witness's testimony.*

The game plan is simple. The prosecutor presents enough evidence to provide "proof beyond reasonable doubt," while the defense counsel will do everything humanly possible to raise doubts, discredit, and refute the prosecution's evidence and approach. Although one is supposedly innocent until proven guilty, Winick indicates that 25 percent of potential jurors initially believe the accused person to be guilty (otherwise why would there be a trial), and 36 percent believe that the defendant is responsible for proving innocence.

As we begin to play the "bullets/bracelets" game as either the accused or as a witness, there are a few basic suggestions which seem to apply in almost every situation:

1. Be honest. Not only is there an ethical responsibility, but when you are honest, you don't have to remember what you said. It should be noted, however, that honesty is relative; how one couches words is extremely important. As an example, *hitting* another car may be viewed quite differently from *smashing* into another car.

2. Admit weakness. State only what you know; neither speculate nor fantasize on the stand. If you do not know, state that you do not know. Brief hesitation, looking puzzled, stammering, etc., may indicate that you don't know what you are talking about.

3. Anticipate questions. Work with your attorney on anticipating questions to minimize surprises. Most certainly, answers to questions from your attorney should be fully discussed, carefully thought out, and possibly rehearsed.

4. Take time to think. Especially when being cross-examined, there is a tendency to try to give quick, rapid-fire responses. If you feel you are losing control or you know the answer but can't quite think of it, say "Let me think about that for just a moment." This is a powerful technique which puts you in control. Silence in a courtroom is devastating and it makes you appear intelligent.

5. Clarify the questions. If the question is not clear, ask that it be repeated or rephrased. Sometimes it is advisable to ask after you have responded, "Did that answer your question?" or "Am I making myself clear?"

Once again, keep in mind that the purpose of the cross-examination is to make the witness appear ignorant, irresponsible, or biased. The witness intellectually "bracelets these bullets" through quiet competence and mastery.

Once you understand that judges, juries, witnesses, attorneys, and defendants are human, you can take a look at how **PeopleWise®** **Motivation** has been used in the courtroom. The situation described earlier about the car pulling out from a roadside service station which resulted in sliding into another vehicle was true. Furthermore, it was serious — the estimated damage to both cars exceeded $10,000. As my attorney and I planned the defense, we decided to prepare two specific approaches — a Level 4 approach for the absolutist-type judge and a Level 5 approach for an aggressive, young, aspiring judge.

The Level 4 approach would be straight forward, matter-of-fact, and presented with sincerity underlined with the theme "give me a break — I'm innocent — I'm not looking for justice — I'm looking for sympathy." The Level 5 approach would be presented in a confident, aggressive, flashy style that would say, "Look, this jerk pulled out in front of me; I'm the good guy; that other unknown person is the bad guy — I want justice."

To prepare for the Level 4 approach, we took eight pictures with a Polaroid camera showing what the highway looked like as we approached the scene of the accident. For this approach, we would plead innocent in a humble, almost embarrassed fashion. When asked to state our case, we would say things like:

"Your honor, I feel very uncomfortable here, but I honestly do not feel I was driving recklessly. Yes, I did hit the car, but there were some extenuating circumstances that, if permitted, I would like to explain. To begin with, it was about 8:15 a.m. and I was heading west on 29 to pick up my friend in Ivy. His truck broke down and he needed a way to school; he teaches special education at Burley. As I was approaching the gas station, a car suddenly pulled out in front of me. I didn't know what to do, so I immediately changed lanes, only to find that a car was stopped waiting to turn left about 20 yards up the highway. Since there wasn't any other lane or place to turn, I slammed on my brakes and slid into the back of the car turning left. The person who pulled out from the gas station didn't stop. I guess they just didn't want to get involved — maybe they were scared or something, I don't know. Judge, I've taken some pictures to show you exactly what happened."

At this point, I would show the pictures and go through the accident in detail. Then I would say, "I don't know the law or anything like that, but I assure you I wasn't speeding, zigging in or out of traffic, or anything like that. I guess you will have to be the judge (laugh a little here). I don't know, I'm just sick about it. Do you have any questions?"

To prepare for the Level 5 approach, we took a videotape of the accident area and additionally recorded the testimony, on an audiotape, of the station attendant verifying that the car pulled out in front of us (taking care not to record that, in the opinion of the station attendant, I was going too fast to stop). For this approach, we would plead innocent in a confident manner. The presentation would go like this:

"Your honor, I fully realize that the situation does not look good for me; however, I am confident I was not driving recklessly. In fact, I think I took every precaution in preventing a serious accident. At 8:15 sharp I was heading west on 29 to pick up a teaching companion of mine. I was going well under the speed limit, of which the skid marks on the pavement will testify. Suddenly, without warning, a car darted out in my pathway from the Shell station on my right. I immediately moved my car left into the inside turning lane, which was the only open lane, to avoid hitting the car. Twenty yards up was another car turning left. I instinctively applied my brakes and, unfortunately, there was some gravel and sand on the road which made me skid into the back of the turning vehicle. Thank God no one was hurt. I didn't have time to get the license number of the car that pulled out, but it was a cream Camaro.

"The next day I went out and took a videotape of the scene of the accident, and I have a recorded testimony of the station attendant verifying that a car pulled out in front of me. I couldn't convince the attendant to come here today, but I do have the station's number. I would be glad to show the video or, if you prefer, I can play the testimonial tape for you. I hope I have been clear in my description of the accident, for I fully believe the darting car caused the accident. Had there been no darting car, there would have been no accident. What questions can I answer that might help you?"

The result was: a Level 4 judge, after a Level 4 presentation, issued a *not guilty decision*. Brain-to-brain makes sense and helps promote justice.

PeopleWise® Motivation also can be used to get a job or be promoted. In real life there are winners and losers, there are those who get promoted and those who don't get promoted, there are those who are employed and those who are unemployed.

In the real world, you don't *almost* win, you don't *almost* get promoted, you are not *almost* employed. Either you are or you aren't.

For those who want to get a job or for those who want to help someone get a job, **PeopleWise® Motivation** can help. An important lesson in life is: *Don't look for complicated answers to simple questions.* Why do some people get jobs and others don't? The answer is simple. They learned how to sell themselves. They convinced an employer they were better than the next person. They sold the employer on the idea that they were a good investment. When I speak of employers, I am talking about the person responsible for hiring, whether it be a personnel manager, employer, or owner. I am referring to the person who has the authority to hire.

I have helped countless people acquire jobs, and have assisted hundreds of placement counselors in the development of skills for placing people in productive employment. I have taken individuals who had many things going against them, people with prison records, people over 50 who had no work record whatsoever, people in their late 40s who had terrible work records with literally not one successful work experience, and people of limited intellectual capacity. I have taken these people and successfully placed them into productive employment. How? By studying and analyzing various hiring procedures and by systematically testing ways to persuade employers to hire my friends, my people, my clients. By implementing **PeopleWise® Motivation** with employers, I have put into practice all we have learned about dealing with people brain-to-brain.

It is true that individual skills affect employability, but after studying thousands of people who just couldn't seem to get a job, it became obvious that these people simply couldn't sell themselves. *These people couldn't get through the interview.* They had developed no interview skills. The solution was to teach them how to sell themselves.

How do you sell yourself? First, you must convince yourself you are worth selling; secondly, you must develop skills in selling yourself.

Everyone has faults. No one is perfect. Every single solitary individual has worth and can be a contributing member in the world of employment. Everyone has something to offer an employer whether it be technical skill, manual labor, ideas, or loyalty. Before you can sell yourself, you must convince yourself that you are worth selling.

I've seen talented individuals convince themselves they aren't worth hiring. I've seen individuals in employment lines with 35 years of successful working experience convinced they have nothing to offer a company or business. I've seen intelligent people with graduate degrees convinced they are dumb. Why do these people rank themselves so low on the self-worth scale? Because they have psyched themselves out, because they have brainwashed themselves, because they have developed the habit of putting themselves down.

It can happen to anyone. Wayne Dyer, in his book, *The Sky's the Limit*, tells the story about a lady in her early forties who constantly puts herself down. It seemed that in the early afternoons she would get so depressed she just couldn't stand herself. Her counselor, her psychologist, her psychiatrist couldn't seem to help her. One day she went to her gynecologist for a checkup. Toward the end of the exam she mentioned how she would get depressed in the afternoon. The physician looked at her in amazement and explained:

This is absurd. Look at you — you are intelligent, you are talented, you are beautiful. Look at that body; you have the body of a 26 year old. Look at your skin; you have the skin of a 23 year old. And look at your breasts; you have the breasts of a 20 year old. The next time you get depressed, take pride in yourself. Stand up and say to yourself, "*I'm attractive, I'm talented, I am beautiful, I like myself.*" If necessary to convince yourself, strip your clothes off and look at yourself in a mirror.

A couple of days later she was cleaning house and, as usual, she felt herself beginning to get depressed. She stopped and immediately stripped off all her clothes. As she stood in front of a mirror, she began rubbing her hands all over her body, admiring the texture of her skin, the shape of her body, and the softness of her hair. Suddenly, without notice, her husband came in and, as he saw her standing in front of the mirror, he questioned, "What are you doing?" She quickly explained what the physician had recommended and then promptly said, as she turned from side to side, "The doctor told me I have the body of a 26 year old and I should be proud." She then began to rub her hands all over her body while her husband looked on. "The doctor said I had the skin of a 23 year old." Her hands moved up her thighs, past her stomach to her chest. She suddenly grabbed both her breasts, held them firmly in her hands, and turned to him. As she faced him she said, "See, these are the breasts of a 20 year old."

In a tone of disgust, the husband quickly responded with, "Did the doctor say anything about your 40-year-old ass?"

As she calmly turned back toward the mirror, she matter of factly retorted, "No, your name was never brought up in the conversation."

You see, she began to realize she had value, she was important, she had worth. One of the sad things in life is that too few people go around complimenting other people. Too few people go around telling you how good you are. Too few people help you determine your strengths.

Each and every person has skills. If you can't think of any of your own, take some time to sit down and list all the things you do throughout an average week. Then list what else you could do. These are skills you have that, when asked, you can be proud to share with a future employer.

After you have convinced yourself you are worth selling, you must develop some skills in selling yourself.

To sell yourself, you must persuade an employer you are better than the other applicants. To sell yourself, you must do so *in person*. No one is hired from a resumé or from a letter of application. Resumés and letters of application are used to stimulate employer interest in you, or possibly, used to test the water to see if there is an opening. Resumés and letters of application need to be clear, neat, accurate, and concise, but the real test comes during the interview. Interviews are used to determine whether you get the job or not. The minute you step into the room, the interviewer begins to form opinions of you; therefore, it is important to be prepared before you get into the room.

Many books have been written about getting a job and all contain some valuable information. However, my experience has shown that if you want to persuade an employer to hire you over someone else, you must do more than conduct yourself well through the interview; you must do more than put your best foot forward; you must do more than answer all the questions correctly; *you must sell yourself.*

Typical types of information that you find in books on how to conduct yourself during an interview emphasize such things as maintain good posture, dress appropriately, act natural, be relaxed, use eye-to-eye contact, answer questions in an organized fashion, don't argue, smile, listen, enunciate distinctly, show interest, thank the interviewer for the time spent with you, etc. Although all these suggestions are well intentioned, the truth is you could do all of these things very well and still not get the job because you didn't sell yourself. Selling yourself is the key. Unfortunately, selling yourself is just as difficult as selling a car, or selling a set of encyclopedias, or selling some waterless cookware, or selling a vacuum cleaner, ... Not only is selling yourself just as difficult, it takes just as much, if not more, skill.

To develop the skills to sell yourself, we must closely analyze the hiring habits of employers — the personnel buying habits, if you please. What do employers look for in an employee? Different employers look for different things. Employers are people and all of the things we learned about people apply to employers. *Everything we learned about* **PeopleWise® Motivation** *directly applies to selling yourself.*

You guessed it; employers fall into predominantly three types: (a) absolutist, (b) materialist, and (c) sociocentric. Let's briefly review them.

Absolutist Employers

Absolutist employers are conservative employers, usually those who are operating their own proprietorships. They have generally pulled themselves up by their own boot straps, and they believe that the way to get ahead is through perseverance (e.g., keeping one's shoulder to the wheel and nose to the grindstone). Often they are family people who have started and developed their businesses primarily for their family. They devoutly believe in the worth of rules and regulations, and they usually run their organizations in an autocratic fashion with many policies and guidelines to be followed. Many times these documents are posted for the employees to see. Their organizations may often be described as rigid, and this characterization is often exemplified by the presence of a time clock which **everybody** punches in and out. Absolutists view themselves as pillars of the community and believe that they have a responsibility to civic organizations and just causes.

Materialistic Employers

Materialistic employers are more cause-and-effect oriented. They are "slicker" (i.e., rather than persevering to get ahead, they are seen as more calculating or manipulative). They believe that it is *who* you know rather than *what* you know that counts. They are production-oriented, make extensive use of charts and graphs, and are usually fairly successful. They like to display themselves through the purchase of expensive watches and portable calculators, by driving large, flashy cars, and by dressing in the latest fashion. On the whole, they look and act just as a sharp business person would be expected to look and act.

Sociocentric Employers

Sociocentric employers are a relatively new breed, having come to the forefront only within the last five to eight years; and, while these individuals are rare, they are quite important. They have usually inherited their businesses from their parents or close relatives. They are not production-oriented, but, rather, people-oriented, believing that the "real" purpose in life is not to make money or develop a large corporation. The real life purpose of sociocentric individuals is to get along with people, to love, to develop friendship. These people, not being obsessed with production, are opposed to competition and just want to get the job done. They build their organization around employees, and their businesses often take on the "one big, happy family" atmosphere. As a matter of fact, the success of the sociocentric employer's organization is often judged by how well his/her employees get along among themselves.

When you apply for a job you will encounter one of the three types of employers (or combination). Keep in mind, they are in the position to do the hiring and it is their responsibility to select the best person for the job. It is your responsibility to convince an employer that you are the best person for the job.

Most interviews start with some small chit-chat to break the ice, so to speak. Common questions are: How are you? What brings you to this particular business? What do you think about the weather? The questions are usually asked out of habit while the employer skims over your completed application or resume. Keep in mind, it is extremely difficult, if not impossible, to sell yourself unless you establish a common bond with the employer. You must get the employer's attention that you are *the* person for the company. *You must establish rapport.*

Professionals who are involved in persuasion, selling, motivation and management know the importance of establishing rapport, but few books or individuals actually teach a person how to develop the skills for establishing rapport. Most professionals assume that you know how important it is to strike a common cord, establish rapport, hit on common ground. Establishing rapport is a lot like shaking hands — everyone knows it is important, and everyone assumes you know how to shake hands. If you have ever shaken hands with someone who didn't know how to perform that act — like shaking a wet fish or holding a limp dish cloth — then you know that a poor hand shake leaves a very bad impression. The truth is, people are not innately skilled in performing many relatively simple tasks that are taken for granted. Establishing rapport falls into this highly neglected category.

Many people are at a loss for words and/or ideas for talking with others. The establishment of rapport involves both listening and talking. The ultimate goal of establishing rapport is *getting the other person to talk about things in which they think you are interested.* That's right, getting the other person to talk while you listen — intently, interestingly, sincerely, captivatingly, acknowledgingly. People like to hear themselves talk. Interviewing people, day in and day out, for jobs is very boring. You would be surprised how many interviewers have a need to break away from their interviewing format to just talk about *something they are interested in.*

Most people are under the misconception that when they talk, they are in control. Listening, asking appropriate questions at the right time, and responding crisply and accurately place an individual in control during an interview. That is correct — listening and keeping quiet places a person in control. Who talks the most on David Letterman's late night talk show, Dave or his guests? You are right, his guests talk much more; Dave listens, asks questions, and occasionally responds. Is there any question who is in control? No, Dave definitely controls the conversation. The same is true for you during an interview. In order to sell yourself you need to gain some control. You gain control by listening, asking good questions, and responding accordingly. Before you can ask good questions, you must know what to listen and look for. Let's take another look at the three types of employers.

Absolutist employers traditionally dress in a conservative fashion. They wear plain brown or black shoes, which may be a little scuffed. If they wear suits, they usually look uncomfortable (these people are pretty easy to pick out in church). Their offices may have a Rotary or Pilot sign or plaque displayed on the wall, generally indicating years of service rendered, because being associated with an organization over time is important to these individuals. They will often have family pictures on their desks so that they may look up from their work occasionally to see them. Of course, these pictures provide one topic of conversation that can be safely broached.

They most likely will explain that the pictures are of a spouse, children, or grandchildren. With a little encouragement, they will tell you everything from soup to nuts about the family. At an appropriate pause, you may wish to pull out your wallet and promptly display your family. You have achieved a common ground — you are, as we say, establishing rapport. Do not feel that you are conning or manipulating this person, because you will enjoy talking about your family just as much as anyone else does. If they don't have a family, talk about the Armed Services since these individuals may have served in some capacity. You might ask what branch of the service they were in, where they were stationed, etc., and share your own experiences. If you haven't been in the service, talk about church, Rotary or Pilot organizations, local politics, etc. Absolutist employers value sincerity, honesty, dedication, loyalty, hard work, sacrifice. Any questions you ask or any responses you make must fit into what an absolutist believes or thinks. *This is establishing rapport, this is selling yourself, this is putting your best foot forward, this is a part of using* **PeopleWise®** **Motivation** *during an interview.*

Spotting **materialistic** employers is fairly easy, since they look like, act like, and have the expectations and needs of our stereotypical, traditional, competitive business person. Their offices will be more plush than those of the absolutists, and if they have a Rotary or Pilot sign or plaque on their wall, it will usually indicate positions held by them in an organization, rather than years of service. If family pictures are present, they will generally be found hanging on the wall rather than sitting on the desk.

Bear in mind that these people want to demonstrate their success and, therefore, they flaunt their accomplishments. For example, the photographs of their families will usually be nicely matted and framed, and ordinarily will project a group portrait. Seldom will these individuals have a polaroid picture of any member of their families taped to their wall or sitting on their desks; polaroid pictures are normally found in the middle drawer of the materialist employer's desk.

These people may not necessarily want to talk about their families, since these are matters remote from business and attaining success. They may, however, wish to talk about their children's accomplishments in school or in local organizations, or about some committees on which they are serving.

One topic of conversation that is almost certain to elicit some response is sports. One can usually get some hints on the preferred sport by looking around the office for trinkets and trophies. If you choose not to talk about these topics, you may wish to talk about the furnishings of the office (especially floor coverings, since these individuals tend to prefer carpeted offices), or possibly about the latest fashion trends. We have found that almost all materialistic employers seem to enjoy talking about shoes. This may sound strange, but these people seem to have an obsession with the topic. Most of them wear well-shined designer shoes and, as you sit in materialist employers' offices, you can't help but notice how they flash these shoes around, lifting their feet, crossing their legs — they just generally seem to be very proud of their shoes. This fetish also carries over to casual wear, where deck shoes and/or expensive running shoes have become in vogue. At any rate, this displaying of shoes happens unconsciously. When one merely comments, "Wow, I sure like those shoes. Where did you get them?" the materialistic employer will begin a short dissertation on their construction, their history and, of course, their cost.

When dealing with materialistic employers, it pays to be aware of the latest fads. Currently to be found on such a list are pinky rings (especially those with a family crest), diamond tennis bracelets, "slide" bracelets, digital watches, pocket calculators, car phones, laptop computers, fax machines, Ping putters, graphite shaft drivers, aerodynamically designed golf balls, and the more advanced of the power-designed composite tennis racquets. Materialistic employers value drive, competitiveness, eagerness, competence, forcefulness, daring, risk-taking, self-assurance, decisiveness, confidence, adventure. All questions and responses should mesh with the materialistic employer's ideas.

Sociocentric employers tend to be more casual in all respects than the absolutist or materialist employer. They generally wear sweaters or sport shirts and seem to like Rockports or other comfortable footwear. In extreme cases, one may find them wearing Birkenstock sandals or thongs. It's almost a sure bet that one is dealing with a sociocentric employer if the person in a hiring capacity isn't wearing socks.

These individuals enjoy talking about people, feelings, fellowship, togetherness, etc. Common topics of conversation are ecology, the ozone layer, global issues, alternate forms of energy, sailing, and bicycling. Their offices often display posters with slogans like "Today is the first day of the rest of your life"; and, of course, it's always a good bet to make some comment on their posters or favorite saying. Sociocentric employers value creativity, nontraditionalism, individuality, freedom, spontaneity, warmth, and friendliness. Most importantly, remember that sociocentric employers take their time in making a decision. You shouldn't apply any pressure whatsoever. They hire those individuals with whom they feel comfortable — from whom they receive good vibes.

So, to sell yourself, you must establish good rapport with your future employer. To establish rapport, you couch your words, phrases, questions, and responses in a language and manner that is compatible with the employer's expectations. I am not in any way recommending that you lie or even color the truth a little. I want to help you understand how employers think and act, and that you can use **PeopleWise®** **Motivation** strategies successfully with a future employer. **PeopleWise®** **Motivation** strategies provide you with a format for dealing with employers in a precise, specific, and effective way.

As you enter the interview, immediately begin sizing up the employer. Don't get anxious. Don't begin to establish rapport until it is convenient to ask questions. Sometimes you can ask a question following one of your responses to a question from the interviewer. As an example, an interviewer, while glancing over your completed application, may comment, "I see from your application that you have two children; what are their ages?" Your response to an absolutist employer might be, "My youngest, Janet, is four and Kim is eight. (Pause) Excuse me, but I couldn't help noticing the pictures on your desk. Are they of your family?"

"Why yes."

"What are their ages?"

"Twelve and fifteen."

"Where do they go to school?" etc.

Same question from a materialistic employer, "I see from your application you have two children, what are their ages?"

"My youngest is Janet, age four, and she is attending Canterbury Nursery School. Kim is eight, she recently was in the school play and she got to introduce each act. We are very proud of her. (pause) Excuse me, I couldn't help noticing the picture on the wall. The girl in the basketball uniform — is she your youngest or oldest?"

"Oldest."

"How long was she a basketball player?" etc.

Same question from the sociocentric, "I see from your application you have two children, what are their ages?"

"My youngest, Janet, is four, and Kim is eight. (brief pause) I couldn't help noticing that picture with the beautiful view. Two years ago when we went hiking in the Sierras, Kim loved it. Do you like to camp out?"

"Why, yes, I do."

"Where was your last trip?" etc.

You get the idea. Get the other person talking about things they think you are interested in hearing.

If you can't conveniently get a question in, don't force it because in every interview, at some time, the employer is going to ask, "Do you have any questions?" NEVER SAY NO! More than 80 percent of job applicants respond that they don't have any questions; *this eliminates any chance to sell oneself.* First, ask a couple of job-related questions, then move into the **PeopleWise**®-type questions that establish rapport. If you have already established good rapport, then move on to some tough interesting questions like:

What are you looking for in an employee?

Why did you, personally, choose this company over another company?

If you could summarize in three to five sentences what this company stands for, what would you say?

Tell me a little about the history of this company; how did it get started?

If you were I, what questions do you think I should be asking that I haven't thought of?

If you don't get a job during the first interview, think about how you handled yourself, how you came across, what questions you could have asked, and specifically about those questions you didn't answer very well. No one is perfect, and some people think better on their feet than others. However, if you write down the questions that you have been asked, after several interviews, you will have built up a list of questions to help you prepare for future interviews. The following are just a few interview questions that sometimes give applicants problems:

How would you describe yourself over the phone to a person who had never met nor seen you?

What do you think will be the most difficult part of the job you are applying for?

What do you have to offer us that someone else doesn't, or why should I hire you over someone else?

What have you done that would convince me you really want to work for our company?

These questions are asked to see how well you can think on your feet. There are no correct answers, but the average applicant doesn't answer them very well.

At the conclusion of the interview, ask when the decision will be made to hire and if you will be notified, regardless of the decision. No matter what the response is, follow-up the interview with a call and/or letter asking if you can provide any more information. Emphasize that you need and want the job and you want to give them anything you can to help them make a decision. Hopefully, the decision will be to hire you.

For just a moment, think about what you need to know just to establish rapport with these three types of employers. It is helpful if you are knowledgeable, or at least able, to talk somewhat intelligently about families, automobiles, bicycles, civic organizations, clothes, pocket calculators, digital watches, pollution, ecology, wall posters, various types of music, computers, cellular phones, global economy, time management, nutrition and exercise, types of wine, specific sports, etc., etc., etc. Learning **PeopleWise® Motivation** skills isn't easy, but once applied, these skills are effective. Dealing with people brain-to-brain and using the mental development staircase is powerful and can benefit anyone in real life, in real situations, in real time. Figure 13-1 places a lot of impor-

	Absolutist	Materialist	Sociocentric
Preferred Approach	Direct	Competent	Trust
Observable Characteristics	Conservative Traditional Orthodox Standard Status quo	Stylish Fashionable In Vogue Popular Trendy	Casual Comfortable Nonchalant Relaxed Informal
Topics and Interests	Family Grandchildren Local Community Events Bowling Fishing Hunting Baseball American Made Sedan Better Homes and Gardens Reader's Digest Family Circle Woman's Day	Clothes Jewelry Gadgets Basketball Football Golf Tennis Sports Car, Luxury Model Vogue House and Garden Elle Sharper Image Catalog	Wildlife Ecology Peace Biking Canoeing Sailing Camping Minivan The Futurist Omni Discover Prevention
Projection (I AM)	Knowledgeable Reliable	Competent Efficient	Trustworthy Patient

tant **PeopleWise®** information on one page. Use it for a quick review from time to time.

Figure 13-1 — Overview of PeopleWise® Motivation

Characteristics for Absolutist, Materialist, and Sociocentric

PART III:
BRAIN TECHNOLOGY
(Self-Empowerment)

CHAPTER FOURTEEN

THE FIRING OF THE BRAIN

During the 60s, for a brief period of time, I traveled as a professional magician. I was billed as the Great Payndini. This was a time when movie theaters played double features on Saturdays. Between shows, theaters would often have some type of entertainment, like a yo-yo demonstration with contest, clown act with jugglers, or a magic show. I traveled from theater to theater in the Midwest. My typical routine consisted of various slight-of-hand tricks with cards, silks, ropes, and balls; some illusions, my two biggest, were sawing a woman in half and floating a lady; and I did some escape work using handcuffs, chains, and a straight jacket. A small part of my act included hypnosis.

As I gained experience, I began to get booked in dinner theaters and night clubs. As I performed before adult audiences, I noticed the hypnosis part of the performance received the greatest attention. Gradually, the hypnosis portion grew to the point that I was billed only as a hypnotist. As a hypnotist, I would stretch subjects between chairs and stand on them, stick pins in their skin, have them sing as small children, or recite nursery rhymes. I would use post-hypnotic suggestion and have them do something like make baby "goo-goo" sounds when I tugged my right ear after they came out of the trance. One part of the act that was interesting to me was when I suggested an ordinary pencil was getting warm and, eventually, hot, how the subjects reacted. However, one evening I got carried away and suggested the pencil was a piece of metal and was turning white hot. Much to my surprise, one of the subjects refused to drop the pencil and the result was a blistered hand. I couldn't imagine the mind being so powerful it could actually cause a physiological reaction to the degree of blistering a person's hand. This scared me because I realized I was dealing with something quite powerful and I could actually hurt someone. I completely stopped performing that night and returned to school to complete my degree in psychology.

When a subject is in a hypnotic trance the suggested words become true statements and at the time the subject behaves in accordance with the perceived beliefs. Thoughts become truths. This is scary, yet when viewed positively, it becomes exciting. The idea behind controlling the activation of the brain uses many of the concepts purported in hypnosis. Hypnosis bypasses the conscious mind and goes directly to the subconscious. In a sense, the uncontrolled subconscious is our slave and when beliefs are consciously controlled, our slave will dutifully obey our every desire.

As I was completing my degree in psychology I was exposed to many theories related to the brain, intelligence, and learning. The many specific theories fascinated me yet, at the same time, overwhelmed me:

J. P. Guilford – model of intellect
Carl Jung – type classification
William James – functionalism
Kurt Lewin – semi-permeable membranes – field theory
Sigmund Freud – unconscious - conscious – psychoanalysis
John B. Watson – behaviorism
B. F. Skinner – stimulus - response – behaviorism
Konrad Lorenz – imprinting
Noam Chomsky – syntactic structures
Francis Galton & John Stuart Mill – nature – nurture
Ivan Pavlov – conditioned reflex – classical conditioning
Edward Thorndike – law of effect
J. B. Wolfe – secondary reinforcement (tokens)
G. Stanley Hall – recapitulation
Edward C. Tolman – cognitive maps
Doman & Delacato – mixed dominance
Albert Bandura – cognitive theory of observational learning
Walter Cannon – homeostasis
Kurt Kaffka, Wolfgang Köhler, Max Wertheimer – Gestalt – whole parts
John Dewey – pragmatism / instrumentalism
J. Ridley Stroop – interference effect
Hippocrates – temperaments
Alfred Binet – mental age
Charles Spearman – small "g" – general intelligence
Louis Thurstone – primary mental abilities

Lewis Terman – intelligence quotient
David Wechsler – verbal and performance skills
Raymond Cattell – fluid intelligence
Norman R. Ellis – stimulus trace
Jean Piaget – cognitive development
Lawrence Kohlberg – stages of moral reasoning
Erik Erikson – stages of psychosocial development
Samuel Kirk – psycholinguistic modalities

The point is, all these ideas/concepts are theories and nothing but theories. **PeopleWise® Motivation** is a compilation of theories, presented in an understandable format. These theories help explain why people behave the way they do, predict what might happen under certain conditions, and possibly how one might go about causing something to happen. Chapters 1-5 presented ideas from the personal development field specifically related to visual imagery and mental rehearsal. This information can be used to explain why some people are more successful than others, under what conditions success and/or failure is realized, and using a series of steps, how success can be accelerated and failure minimized. Chapters 6-13 presented a developmental theory of psychological growth that proceeds up an ascending staircase leading to predictable landings. This information can be used to explain why some people behave differently than others, when and under what conditions certain behaviors can be anticipated, and how to use the information to assist others in their learning, growth, development, and maturation. This chapter introduces ideas/concepts related to the firing of the brain, sometimes referred to as brain activation. Understanding brain activation is simple but the implications are of the highest magnitude.

Instruments exist that somewhat accurately measure the activation impulses of the brain. Simply stated, electrodes that measure electrical current (brain waves) are attached to the outside of the head. These instruments provide information that suggest that in most people, most of the time, the activation in the brain is scattered. However, when a person begins to concentrate or focus on something with a high degree of intensity, the activation of the brain becomes more localized in a specific section of the brain. When the concentration or focus becomes so intense the individual enters a high state of consciousness known as the "zone" or "flow," the activation becomes pinpointed in a relatively small area. The "zone" or "flow" activation area is always small, but varies in locations from person to person, i.e., in some individuals the localization occurs predominately on the left side, others, on the right, and still others in the front or rear. People can be taught how to control this brain activation. In other words, people can be taught how to improve their concentration and focus which, in turn, improves their performance. This is easily demonstrated when improving one's development in a specific physical skill, like shooting a basket, putting, hitting, or kicking a ball. The controlling of brain activation is applicable for pitching horseshoes, throwing darts, singing, running a marathon, conducting a meeting, getting along socially with others, speaking before an audience, meditating, studying, or creating.

The control of the firing of the brain is the key that unlocks the door to the subconscious. Consider for a moment the two functions of the subconscious: automatic and learned. The automatic function happens without thought: heartbeat, circulation, breathing, digestion, and other bodily functions. The learned function takes over automatically as a habit is formed: tying shoes, walking, speaking, memorizing, driving, riding a bicycle, adding, subtracting, multiplying, dividing, reading, etc.

Take something for granted, like catching a ball. The brain has to do a lot of complex things for a successful catch. Now complicate the matter by having the person run to get to the ball to catch it. Now distract the person by having people yell and scream. Finally, fill the subconscious with degrading comments to the point the person believes they are of little worth and they are unsuccessful and they can't do anything right. When an individual gets into the "zone," they are able to screen out all the junk and screen in only those things that are necessary for a successful catch and they do this unconsciously. The goal is to achieve Olympian focus. Olympian focus just doesn't happen. Olympian focus is learned by influencing the subconscious through the controlling of the firing of the brain.

During brain surgery, studies report that patients whose brain cells are stimulated with thin electrodes describe reliving scenes from the past. Keep in mind, they are not remembering, they are reliving the experiences. When you control the firing of the brain, you experience sensations that allow you to "post-live." In other words, you create the future rather than relive the past. When you "post-live," you experience whole heartedly before it happens — you "will" it to happen. People who get into the "zone" are actually post-living, that is, they are seeing, feeling, and experiencing the future event before it happens. In other words, they create the future.

Most scientists today agree that the functions of the brain cannot be simply compartmentalized as right or left brain dominant. Functions frequently appear in both hemispheres at the same time, but for most people the right side of the brain seems holistic, intuitive, and nonverbal while the left appears temporal, analytic, and verbal.

Researchers Amy Haufler and Bradley Hatfield, in their video tape, *Math Like You Have Never Seen It Before*, narrated by Danny Glover, contend the left side of the brain is verbal, the right side is space and movement, the front is emotional and the rear is visual. They have studied skilled and novice rifle shooters. By placing electrodes on the skull they measure brain waves simultaneously with the accuracy of rifle shots. Basically, they have concluded: novice shooters' brain activation is scattered, skilled shooters' brain activation is localized, and in Olympian shooters, five seconds before trigger pull, the firing of the brain is even more pinpointed than in skilled shooters, indicating superior focus and concentration. By demonstrating to shooters how the brain activation relates to the accuracy of the shots, improvement in shooting is experienced. In other words, as one trains the body, one trains the mind. By utilizing visual imagery/mental rehearsal and the developmental staircase, with what we know about brain activation, we can reverse the process — as one trains the mind, one trains the body.

You start to learn a physical skill through trial and error. You usually learn a few basics then you practice, practice, practice. As you get better, it becomes a habit. The habit is predominantly controlling the learned function of the subconscious. What separates the good player from the excellent player is mostly mental. The excellent player just seems to "will" it to happen. Also, the excellent player doesn't let failures bother them as much as the good player.

You are shooting a free throw and you are doing well. All of a sudden, you shoot an air ball. When you get ready to shoot after the air ball, it is hard to get the bad shot out of your mind. You keep mentally seeing the ball missing the rim and you imagine people laughing at you, so you try to **consciously** force or guide the shot. What has happened is the subconscious has taken hold of you and the only thing you think you can control is the conscious part of your brain. The subconscious always wins over the conscious. Same thing with golf. You miss a putt and all of a sudden you get the "yips." You try to **consciously** guide or force the ball in the hole. Same with bowling or hitting a ball, or fouling up on an interview or missing a sale. It is all the same, the subconscious controls our behavior as we try to out conscious the subconscious.

Or you have a successful string going and you realize you are going to set a personal best. All of a sudden you get overly anxious, overly sensitive, overly everything. What has happened is the subconscious has taken over to tell you enough is enough.

What we know now goes beyond visual imagery and mental rehearsal. We know we can go directly to controlling the firing of our brain and control the subconscious by realizing where our brain fires naturally. Level 4s fire on the left, 5s on the right, 6s in the front and 7s in the rear. Each Level utilizes visual imagery and mental rehearsal differently. The principles we learned in Chapters 1-5 in personal development are the same, but the actual execution varies. The ascending staircase tells us how to execute the activity, in other words, how we go about learning to control the firing of our brain at Levels 4, 5, 6, and 7. Levels 1, 2, and 3 are still at the reactive stage and proactive control of the subconscious is not possible. I remember, during a training session conducted by Clare Graves, he showed two slides of slices of brain cells, one from a schizophrenic who died in an institution and the other taken from a cat. The cell structures of the two were indistinguishable from one another. His point was, lower-level brains have less fire power than upper level brains. We take what we know from personal development and the ascending mental staircase and we apply what we have learned from brain activation, which is, just prior to getting in the "zone," the firing of the brain becomes pinpointed. Theoretically, the pin-pointedness is directly related to the landings on the mental staircase. Now, for the first time in the history of humankind, we know how to improve our skill development by directing the firing of our brain, which gives us control of our subconscious. There may be other ways to improve skill development, but **PeopleWise® Motivation: The Art of Motivating Brain-to-Brain** is the most direct, most systematic, most comprehensive, and the most powerful.

CHAPTER FIFTEEN

Skill Development Like You've

Never Thought of Before

once had an opportunity to advise a discus thrower on the track team at the University of Virginia. He came to me because in practice he performed extremely well, but during a meet he seemed to choke up and fouled constantly. A **PeopleWise**® analysis found that he was a Level 6 who was practicing like a Level 4. He had a favorite discus (Level 4 thinking) and he carried it everywhere with him. He felt this discus was a part of him, sort of an extension of his body. This type of thinking is healthy for a Level 4, but a Level 6 who gets a favorite discus begins to get the idea that a great deal of the distance thrown is related to the discus itself. Sure enough, I found that when given two other identical discuses, he always threw his favorite discus the farthest.

My job was simple. I had to convince him that he was the important element in the process of throwing the discus. I did this by taking his favorite discus away and providing him with three identical discuses of different colors: one red, one orange, and one blue. Each day, he would throw each discus three times, with all distances recorded. Afterwards, he would practice as usual, but not with his favorite discuss. Over a period of three weeks he was shown that no particular discus was superior. In other words, I wanted him to realize that he was in complete control of throwing the discus — the discus itself was irrelevant. I wanted him to build confidence in himself to such a degree that he would know *he could throw* any discus, rock, hammer or plate farther than anyone.

As he began to realize that his personal talent was responsible for his success, he was given his favorite discus back. He quickly found that he threw it as far but no farther than the others. He won the next meet, set two school records and, most importantly, he never fouled once for the rest of the season.

Obviously I was working with a very talented athlete who had superior physical talent, but for some reason, became distracted or would psych himself out during a meet. He was psychologically, emotionally, and intellectually healthy and if it were legal to count or measure his performance in practice, without competition, he would not have needed any motivational help. However, when he was in a meet he would put pressure on himself and just prior to throwing the discus he would consciously try to control his focus but his subconscious would override the conscious and distract him to such a degree he would choke up and foul. In other words, his subconscious was leading him to the rock in the road. When I discovered he had Level 6 tendencies, theoretically, his brain would naturally fire in the front part, but he practiced as a Level 4 using rigid repetition with the same discus, forcing his brain to fire in the left hemisphere. Thus, during a meet when it was paramount to optimize the firing of the brain in a small localized area to obtain Olympian focus, he couldn't do it because the brain wanted to fire in the front but he was forcing it to fire on the left side.

Whenever there is a battle between the conscious and the subconscious, the subconscious always wins. In his case, when the discus thrower didn't put pressure on himself he had great concentration. Over time, by practicing like a Level 4 through rigid, rigorous, persevering repetition, he learned to fire his brain in the left hemisphere. However, when the pressure was on, the front part of his brain competed with the left, thus he became distracted because his brain could not screen out all the junk that was going on around him. By forcing him to practice using the front part of the brain, which was natural to him (being a Level 6), he became more confident in himself because the brain was firing more naturally. The result was, when the pressure was on, the brain fired wholeheartedly in the front without competition from the left hemisphere, thus extraneous junk was screened out and the firing of the brain became pinpointed in the front, creating Olympian focus.

Using standard visual imagery and mental rehearsal techniques, as explained in Chapters 1-5, it would have been possible to override the natural tendency for the front part of the brain to fire; however, this would have taken extraordinary time, energy and practice. By using **PeopleWise®** **Motivation** we are able to short circuit the process and get results quicker, faster, and with less effort. Brain-to-brain motivation doesn't try to make water run up hill. When using **PeopleWise®** **Motivation**, instead of trying to force the process, we let the process happen naturally and effortlessly. **PeopleWise®** **Motivation** will not work by making a strained, conscious effort. The secret of motivating brain-to-brain is to determine where the brain wants to fire most naturally and then align the practice methods accordingly.

I used a similar strategy with a golfer when her putting went sour. This golfer had tendencies to be a 7. After learning about **PeopleWise®** **Motivation**, she described golf as a multi-leveled game. She had determined that driving and long iron shots were Level 5 techniques, mid-irons were Level 4, while short irons and putting strokes were Level 6 techniques. She stated that golf is such a difficult game to master because psychologically you have to switch your mental preparation numerous times from 4 through 6.

She improved her putting (while practicing) by never putting a ball the same distance with the same club. She would use three different putters on the practice green. As she putted six practice balls, she would alternate her putters and, as mentioned earlier, she never putted a ball the same direction or distance. She claimed that a professional putter must develop a feel and sense for putting, so that when she is on the green she is confident that she can get the ball close to, if not in, the hole. Furthermore, a professional putter knows she can hit it with any putter or, as explained in Chapter 1, with a Dr. Pepper bottle. Good putters master touch and feel — they exploit the Level 6 in themselves. A professional golfer does not have to be a Level 7. This Level 7 had simply viewed the game from a **PeopleWise®** **Motivation** standpoint and improved her putting by bringing out the 6 in herself.

A typical Level 4 approach to golf would be Tommy Armour's *How to Play Your Best Golf All the Time*. In this classic book, one finds many rules regarding how to stand, how to hold your elbow, etc. Most of the rules are numbered or are presented in lists. On the other hand, many of the tips on golfing found in *Golf Digest* appeal to Level 5s. Here we find suggestions from professionals that incorporate a cause and effect approach to understanding the game by looking at the swing in terms of weights, balances, arcs, and torque. We find Level 5 discussions on compression and the science of what happens to the ball on contact. The many product changes using different metals and aerodynamic designs are outgrowths of Level 5 thinking.

Level 6s enjoy playing golf, but most do not take the game seriously. Many are not competitive; they have been known to play a round barefooted; and they like to look at the beauty of the landscaping and breathe the clean air. Most 6s are good putters. Level 4s have a regimented approach to the game and play one shot at a time. Level 5s plan a strategy for playing a round as well as a strategy for hitting the ball, while Level 6s just like being outdoors. Often Level 5s take pride in how fast they play a round — they've decided that it is a game of speed. Level 5s enjoy hitting into a foursome of 6s. The 6s enjoy the scenery and, when pushed on the golf course, exhibit a little passive resistance — that is, they intentionally slow down just enough to make things really unpleasant for the people behind them. As a result, the 5s hit into them; the 6s get mad and scream a little; then the 5s grumble and curse while they drive their cart past them. All in all, it seems to be good therapy; everyone's pent-up hostile aggressions are released; and there is an element of psychological healthiness involved in yelling at those you don't know.

The previous paragraph is somewhat sarcastic and written for the most part jokingly, tongue-in-cheek, but, in reality, it isn't too far off from the truth. After testing and interviewing more than 100 weekend golfers, I have found that different **PeopleWise®** Levels exhibit specific habits, characteristics, beliefs, and behaviors directly related to their Level. I determined each golfer's Level of functioning by administering the **PeopleWise® Profile System** similar to the instrument presented in the next chapter, Chapter 16. I asked each golfer to give me words that would describe them and I validated the words with descriptions given to me by their competitors and partners. I observed their play and talked with them about how they approached the game, their beliefs and philosophies, and historically, how they got started.

Left Brain Dominant, Level 4, Absolutist

Disciplined	Regimented
Methodical	Hard on Self
Persistent	Steady
Controlled	Single-Minded

Practice using the same technique over and over and over until your hands get numb. Practice makes perfect. Looking for "the" method or technique. Methodical approach, incremental, step-by-step.

Moe Norman, the founder of Natural Golf, has been classified as a savant of golf. He has earned the reputation of being the best ball striker in the history of the game of golf. He developed his own technique of hitting the ball the same way each and every time, much like a machine. After watching him play for more than two years (never being out of the fairway) an observer noticed he had used the same tee. When asked, "Do you realize you've used the same tee for two and a half years?" his reply was, "Aren't you supposed to?"

In July 2001, I was attending my first Natural Golf Clinic in New Orleans. It was a beautiful day. The air smelled crisp and clean and the temperature was perfect. I was waiting with three other students outside the club house. We knew a little about Moe Norman from a television infomercial and we were anxious to learn this new simplified way of hitting a golf ball. The Master Instructor, Tom Sanders, was a protegé of Moe Norman and had an excellent reputation of being a lot like Moe and an expert ball striker himself. I'll never forget meeting Tom for the first time. He came around the corner of the club house dragging his bag of clubs. He was sort of pear-shaped, his cap was on crooked, and his shirttail was out on the left-hand side. He introduced himself and promptly led us to the driving range, where there were four piles of balls. Each pile could easily have filled one-half of a fifty-five gallon drum barrel. I'd never seen so many balls in one place. He teed up two balls, pointed to the 200-yard sign, and announced he was going to hit the sign. He addressed the ball, looked at the sign, looked down at the ball and, without any hesitation, swung and the ball bounced off the metal 200-yard sign with a loud bang. Before we could say anything, he struck the second ball and it hit the sign with a "ker-thunk." The four of us, speechless, looked at each other in awe. Tom looked up at us and realized something was going on and asked, "Is there something wrong?" One of the students spoke out, saying, "We've never seen that done before." Tom, the Master Instructor, looked at us matter-of-factly and uttered, "Well, it's a pretty big sign."

Next he showed us the baseball grip, how to swing (somewhat like hitting a hockey puck) and how to place the ball in the middle of our stance. For the next three hours, non-stop, we hit balls. Tom moved from student to student, saying the same thing over and over, while the attendant kept us in balls, lots of balls. We took 30 minutes for lunch and returned to hit balls for three more hours without break one. Regardless of club selection, your grip never changed, your swing never changed, and the ball placement never changed. That, my friends, was the clinic. This was a pure Level 4 clinic, conducted by a Level 4 instructor, using a Level 4 process with a Level 4 philosophy. Instead of hitting balls 'til our hands got numb, we hit balls 'til they bled, and then we continued to hit balls while they kept bleeding.

Right Brain Dominant, Level 5, Materialistic

Assertive	Confident
Competitive	Bold
Doer	Decisive
Hard Driving	Aggressive

A student of the game. An avid reader of golf magazines and subscriber to the golf channel. Understands the strategies and physics of the game. Practice doesn't make perfect; perfect practice makes perfect. Attacks the course with a win at all costs attitude. Adrenalin charged using a grip-it and rip-at-it style.

Dave Pelz, president and founder of the Dave Pelz Short Game School, has established himself as the authority of understanding and teaching how to putt and hit short irons. My first Pelz Short Game Clinic took place in Tampa Bay, Florida, at the Westin Innisbrook Resort. The facilities were breathtaking. The morning started in an elegant conference room overlooking the golf course right after a complete breakfast with all the trimmings. There were four instructors that eventually broke us up into three groups of six students. The head instructor laid out the day's agenda and began to show statistics verifying the importance of the short game. Next — through the use of flip charts and graphics — tricks of the short game trade were explained and demonstrated, followed by each group going to the course to begin practicing. Each group went to a separate learning station, i.e., pitch, chip, and sand. The groups rotated every 30 minutes. Teaching aids were used throughout like a bunkerboard for hitting out of sand. The bunkerboard was beveled in the middle, placed in the sand, and a small mound of sand was put on the board with the ball placed on the mound of sand. With little practice you could hit under the ball and guide the ball onto the green. How the club hit the sand to make the ball explode out onto the green was explained much like a lab technician would explain a science experiment in a physics course. Lunch was elegant and very tasty. Following lunch we were introduced to Perfy, the putting robot. Perfy was used to show the physics of striking the ball perfectly. Next, we were introduced to the putting track, which helped monitor the exact pathway of the putter head from take away to follow through. From the putting track we moved to the truthboard. The truthboard had a mirror placed directly behind the ball. When you addressed the ball you should be able to see your eyes in the mirror since good putters have their head directly over the ball — pretty clever and pretty 5ish.

This clinic had more gimmicks than it had students and the instruction was top-drawer. At the end of the clinic, I had more tricks than I had as a traveling magician in the 60s. It was a pure Level 5 clinic, using Level 5 teaching aids by Level 5 instructors in their Level

5 color-coordinated golfing outfits. It was impressive, to say the least.

Forebrain Dominant, Level 6, Sociocentric

Social	Casual
Tolerant	Caring
Patient	Companion
Relaxed	Non-assertive

Golf is primarily for recreation and socialization. While golfing take time to appreciate the environment, nature, and friends. The most important thing in golf is to enjoy and have fun as opposed to winning or beating someone. For the serious Level 6 player, golf is a game of touch, feel, and finesse.

The most unusual golf clinic I ever attended was advertised as "The Inner Game of Golf." The instructor was in his 50s, about 6-feet tall, his hair hung to his shoulders and he was dressed in a short-sleeved, brightly decorated, Hawaiian shirt, jeans, docksiders, and no socks. It took place in Biloxi, Mississippi at the old D'Iberville Hotel. There were only two other participants and myself. As part of the enrollment fee, we received M. Scott Peck's book, Golf and the Spirit. The theme throughout the day was, Golf is a Game of Life Where We Learn About Our Inner Strength.

The session started with all of us removing our shoes and socks. We sat on the floor and we began to learn how to lower anxiety through proper breathing exercises. We would inhale through our nose, hold for six seconds, and exhale through our mouth while touching the tip of our tongue to the upper back of our front teeth. It sounds crazy, but after about ten deep inhales with forced exhales, I began to get light-headed and somewhat dizzy. Next, we did some stretching exercises.

After getting loosened up, each participant shared times while playing golf that were aggravating, unpleasant, and stressful. This was followed by a lecturette on our freedom to choose to be angry or not angry, frustrated or not frustrated. It was explained that no golf ball, golf event, or golf situation could make a person angry unless the individual allowed it to make them angry. We can choose to allow ourselves to be angry or not angry.

Next, we began to explore ways to proact as opposed to react to various golfing situations that might trigger frustration. We looked at various ways to play the game that might lower anxiety, like play a scramble — team plays each player's best ball; provide multiple mulligans to even skill levels; keep a total group score and set a goal to lower the group score by so much within a certain length of time as opposed to keeping individual scores. We learned how to assess the value of play by asking a series of questions after each round like:

Did I win?

Did I try my hardest?

Did I control my thoughts and actions?

Did I have fun?

Did I learn anything?

The idea was, even if a person doesn't win, golf has a lot to offer.

Toward the middle of the afternoon, we were introduced to a blind person who demonstrated his ability to putt. The putting took place in the back of the conference room on the carpet. A cup was rigged up like you might find in someone's office. Even though he couldn't see he was an excellent putter as long as he was told where and how far the cup was and, of course, when he missed, where the ball ended up. We were taught that when the blind use a mobility walking cane they actually sense the tip of the cane as if it were an extended finger.

Each of us was blindfolded and taught the basics of mobility training using a cane and getting a feel for the tip as we tapped around the room. Next, the putter was substituted for the cane as we moved about the room. Finally, the blindfolds were removed and after some brief instruction on putting, we began to learn how to lag to a line, putt through a bridge made of play logo blocks, and finally, into the rigged-up cup. We were all surprised at how our putting improved as we learned to view the putter as an extension of our hands and fingers.

Although the clinic was more like a workshop, it definitely was conducted like a Level 6 program, by a Level 6 instructor, with a Level 6 theme running throughout the day.

Rearbrain Dominant, Level 7, Cognitive

Innovative	Flair
Adventuresome	Joust & Joke
Fearless	Experiment
Inquiring	Aura

Self-evaluation of performance is unrelated to the score. One may evaluate performance as very good, yet score poorly, or one may evaluate performance as terrible, yet beat everybody and score extremely well. Talk to self and then answer back. Adjusts rapidly during a game. When hot, will run a birdie-streak like a professional.

Out of the 100+ samples I interviewed, I only ended up with four individuals whom I could identify as Level 7s. Each one reported having more than two holes in one. Every hole in one was reported as happening on a misty day and they felt strange, as if they were a different person, as if someone inside of them hit the ball in the hole. All reported from time to time they tried to hit the ball differently, like step into the ball like a batter in baseball, run and hit the ball, double swing in two full circles before hitting the ball, hit the ball from a crouched-down position as opposed to standing upright position. All four Level 7 golfers had single-digit handicaps, but they didn't play regularly, once a week at best.

I've never been to a Level 7 golf clinic and I've never heard of one, but I imagine the new millennium will bring Level 7 golfers with Level 7 approaches to the game. When it happens, I imagine they will not look like golfers, play like golfers, or act like golfers, but they will revolutionize the game as we know it today.

Now is the time we separate the wheat from the chaff. We are going to take everything we have learned up to this point and I'm going to put it into a procedure that will allow you to control the firing of your own brain. As you attain the skill of firing your own brain you will develop

Olympian confidence and focus that will improve any physical skill you choose.

Brain science is new. We have learned more about the brain in the past five years than in the past 100. Historically, nearly 90 percent of all neuroscientists are alive today. It is always tempting to take research findings out of context and look for simplistic solutions to complex problems. **PeopleWise® Motivation** will be viewed by some as an over simplification of hemispheric dominance. Keep in mind, **PeopleWise® Motivation** is a theory and not necessarily the truth. However, you can test this theory to determine if it works for you. I will present the procedure for applying **PeopleWise® Motivation** in a format that is understandable and immediately applicable and then I will show you a way to test the theory to determine if it works for you. The genius of **PeopleWise® Motivation** is in its simplicity and the beauty is in its direct usage. Some claim there are no quick fixes, but **PeopleWise® Motivation** is so powerful you will see improvement in your skill development in less than a month. The improvement is visible and measurable.

PeopleWise® Motivation relies heavily on two assumptions: (a) the brain is physiologically effected by the environment and (b) emotion plays a major role on the impact of the brain. Ronald Kotulak, in his book *Inside the Brain*, uses a metaphor of a banquet to illustrate the interaction of the brain and the environment.

"The brain gobbles up the external environment through its sensory system and then reassembles the digested world in the form of trillions of connections which are constantly growing or dying, becoming stronger or weaker depending on the richness of the banquet."

PeopleWise® Motivation feeds the brain highly specialized nutritious environmental food, which super-charges its firing in specified targets. This ultimately leads to Olympian confidence and focus. Marian Diamond introduced the concept of "neural plasticity." Neural plasticity is the brain's ability to constantly change its structure and function in response to external experiences. To assist in structurally altering the brain, **PeopleWise® Motivation** supplies a steady stream of environmental vitamins that enhance localized explosions and reduces randomized and scattered firing of the brain. The brain is essentially curious and

157

PeopleWise® **Motivation** capitalizes on this curiosity by helping the brain make connections between the unknown, to the known — between the attempt, to successful skill execution.

The brain is strongly influenced by emotion. Daniel Goleman's *Emotional Intelligence* and Joseph LeDoux's *The Emotional Brain* have helped us understand the role of emotion on learning. Simply stated, the stronger the emotion connected with an experience, the stronger the memory of the experience. Add emotion into learning and the brain deems the information more important and retention is increased. **PeopleWise®** **Motivation** uses the "emotional key" to unlock the subconscious. In skill development, the subconscious always wins out over the conscious. The trick to firing your own brain is to unlock the subconscious so you control it and it doesn't control you.

Why is it that during the last two minutes of a football game the offense seems to play with greater intensity and concentration? Why is it that during the last 30 seconds of a basketball game, the percentage of completed shots substantially increases from the previous part of the game? Might it not be that the players are more focused, more excited, more **emotional**. What is causing the emotion? Is it the environmental circumstances, like the fans are yelling louder, the clock is ticking, the coach and players are in unity as to exactly what **must** be done, the heart is pumping faster, the adrenalin is flowing more freely ... When the touchdown is made and/or the basketball rips the net, does it take longer to quiet down? Just maybe, **emotion** plays a significant role in getting the brain to fire in a small localized part of the brain that enhances an individual's concentration and focus. What **PeopleWise®** **Motivation** does, it allows you to control the emotion rather than wait for the environment to capture it. When you take charge of injecting emotional probes into your brain you control the firing, but as we learned from Clare Graves, not all emotional probes are the same for everyone. **PeopleWise®** **Motivation** allows us to determine which emotional probe stimulates our brain the best.

Here is where the rubber meets the road. I'm going to lay out the procedure for firing your own brain. Anyone that plays golf knows that games are won and lost on the putting green, yet the average player will not practice putting for any given length of time. Players will endlessly hit balls on a driving range or even chip and pitch, buckets of balls, on a green or at a target, but they won't devote even a quarter of the time to putting.

We know that basketball games are won and lost from the free-throw line, yet it is like pulling teeth to get players to seriously practice shooting free throws. Players will play one-on-one and shoot horse until they are exhausted, but put them on a free-throw line to practice shooting free throws and they are ready to go to the shower.

Why is it that something as important as putting and shooting free throws is so distasteful? Because it is **boring**, that's why. Keep in mind, it is easy to get someone to do something they want to do, but **PeopleWise® Motivation** gets people to do things they don't want to do and, at the same time, somewhat like it. If I can write the rest of this chapter on two of the most boring things in the world and get you to read it, then you can do it, you can practice it, and eventually master it. Why both, putting and shooting free throws, and not just one? By presenting two different activities you will see similarities between the two and it will make it easier for you to generalize to other activities, like throwing darts, pitching horseshoes, shooting pool, bowling, kicking/hitting/throwing a ball, selling a car, presenting at a meeting, speaking before a large audience, and possibly improving a person's writing, spelling, reading and computational skills. **PeopleWise® Motivation** has a broad range of application; it has breadth and depth.

As I show you how to control the firing of your own brain, I assume you have reasonable coordination and you have somewhat mastered the basics. For instance, in free-throw shooting your posture and stance are reasonable, you have the strength to get the ball to the basket, the ball rolls off your fingertips and has a reverse spin vertical to the basket. In putting, you have a comfortable stance, your putter moves relatively straight-through along the aimline, the putter head is perpendicular to the aimline, and you hit the ball on the sweet-spot of the putter. To make **PeopleWise® Motivation** work, you don't have to be a professional, you just need to be able to reasonably execute the skill.

Left Brain Dominant, Level 4, Absolutist

Your strength lies in perseveration, methodical approach, incremental steps, step-by-step process. You will use a SEE-DO process.

In basketball, after you see the ball swish-rip the cords, you get a little excited. Sometimes you even feel a tingling sensation on the back of your neck. What is giving you this momentary emotional high is the ball going through the basket. The challenge is for you to control your emotion so you can inject it into your brain just prior to execution. The more confident you are, the greater the chance you will execute the skill correctly and accurately giving positive results. You are confident when you know you are going to be successful. You gain confidence by seeing yourself and experiencing the feeling of success before you execute. You approach the free throw line with your stance exactly like you want it, you grip the ball in your fingertips exactly like you want it, and you look at the basket and focus on the rim exactly the way you want. Before shooting, you will assist your brain in firing in the left hemisphere. You get your brain to fire in the left hemisphere by visually imagining the ball ripping the net and then sense the emotion of successfully completing the shot. The secret is feeling the tingling sensation **before** you release the ball. The greater you generate this feeling, the more you assist your brain in firing.

As you feel the tingling sensation of swishing the ball, you now release the ball. When the ball goes in, your mind will do a double explosion of excitement and make an imprint on your subconscious. As you repeat this process over and over, you will master mind control by effecting the firing of the brain. Using this process, when you miss the shot you must get the missed thought and feeling out of your mind immediately. When you miss, you will experience a down feeling and it is important to flush that down feeling out of your mind because it will negatively influence your next shot. You flush it out by saying out loud or to yourself, "That's not like me, that's not the Olympian I know I am." One flush is enough. Next, you go back through the process again and you imagine in your "mind's eye" the ball ripping the cords.

If you are less than a 60 percent shooter, move the target closer to you, because if you are below 60 percent your actions will speak louder than your thoughts and pretty soon you will have talked your brain into failure rather than success.

As a Level 4, the most difficult thing for you will be to wait and catch that tingling feeling of success before you release the ball. You are so regimented in your habits, you will have a tendency to go through the motions over and over again, but to control your brain, you must force yourself to feel the success before execution.

SEE — You mentally see and hear the ball go through the basket, which sends emotion through your body and after experiencing the tingling feeling you DO — by releasing the ball.

As a putter, you place the ball about three feet from the cup. You grip the club exactly the way you want, you address the ball exactly the way you want, you look at the cup and then refocus on the ball. You imagine the ball dropping into the cup. Just as the free throw shooter hears the rip of the cords, you hear the plunk of the ball dropping into the bottom of the cup. At this point you experience joy and a tingling sensation. After reveling in the successful experience you strike the ball. As the ball drops in, you get a double charge of emotion. When you miss, flush it out of your mind quickly and begin again. When you practice, make sure you are at a distance where you are at least 60 percent successful. As you control the firing of your brain in the left hemisphere you will improve your skill. When you get at 90 percent plus accuracy, move back six inches. When you get at the distance when it is unreasonable to make the ball go into the hole, make the hole bigger by drawing a chalk line around the hole. Now your target is to get within the chalk line. For the average player, you enlarge the hole by two inches when you get beyond seven feet. At 15 to 20 feet, mentally shoot for getting the ball inside the leather and beyond twenty feet get the ball within one club-length around the hole.

SEE — you mentally see the ball go into the hole and hear the plunk as it drops to the bottom of the cup which sends joy throughout your body and, after experiencing the tingling feeling, you DO — by striking the ball.

Using the SEE-DO process, making sure you feel the emotion before executing the skill, you will experience success that can be objectively determined within less than a month's practice of only thirty minutes a day. If you do not experience improvement, then you either cannot generate the necessary emotional excitement prior to execution or you are not a Level 4.

Right Brain Dominant, Level 5, Materialistic

Your strength lies in your cause and effect type of thinking and your intense drive to make it happen. You will use a TUBE process. By using the TUBE process you will trick your brain into firing in the right hemisphere by being logical and cognitive.

In basketball you would rather do anything but shoot free throws, yet your brain activates in such a way you can learn to control the firing of your brain very quickly and improve your free throw shooting with minimal effort and practice. For you, practice doesn't make perfect, perfect practice makes perfect or perfect practice makes permanent.

Most Level 5s think they are smarter than the coach. To control the firing of your brain, you need to convince yourself you are smarter than you think you are. My job is to show you how to tap into your intelligence. To convince Level 5 players the power of their own brain I have them shoot regular free throws from the free throw line and record the percentage of successful shots made. Next, I move the free-throw line just behind the baseline, the exact same distance from the goal. I have them shoot free throws from this new location and I record the percentage of the made shots. Much to their surprise, Level 5s always shoot a higher percentage from the new location on the side of the basket even though it is the same distance from the goal. I have done this many times with Level 5s and they always, I repeat, always, shoot a higher percentage. (Please note: Level 4s do not shoot a higher percentage from this location; they usually shoot a lower percentage.) I show the Level 5s the data and then I ask, "Why did you shoot a higher percentage from the side of the basket than you did from the front of the basket?" As smart as Level 5s are, they usually can't figure it out and want to try it again. So, I let them do it again. They shoot from the front and then move to the side and, again, I compare the percentages and the side always wins.

Although I am tempted to tell them why they shoot a higher percentage from the side, I dare not. Because if I **tell** them, their immediate brain reaction is to challenge me or question my authority. Thus, if I let them figure it out they don't have to use all that subconscious mental energy to outsmart me. To avoid any subconscious mental confrontation I just have them go to the regular free throw line and, as they shoot, I have them orally, out loud, tell me what is going through their mind. It goes something like this:

"I bounce the ball a couple of times to get loosened up. Sort of get the feel of the ball. One toe is on the line, the other is matched up to my instep, both parallel to one another and perpendicular to the basket. The ball is on my finger tips, I hold it chest high as I focus on the rim. I take dead aim and fire." We go through the procedure a couple of times for elaboration purposes, then we move to the side.

"I bounce the ball a couple of times to get loosened up. Sort of get the feel of the ball. One toe is on the line, the other is matched up to my instep, both parallel to one another and perpendicular to the basket. The ball is on my finger tips, I hold it chest high as I focus on the upper side of the backboard."

"Hold it," I say. "Why the upper side of the backboard and not the rim?" I ask.

"Because I want the ball to just barely pass by the upper side of the backboard, I use the backboard as a guide ... I get it, the guide is closer to me than the basket. I've actually moved the rim a foot to a foot and one-half closer to me. When the basket is closer, my percentage of made shots increases.

Bingo, when you move your focus closer, the basket moves closer (for Level 5s). Much like pin bowling vs. spot bowling. When bowling, one learns there are spots about a third of the way down the alley. When you release the ball the same way from the same position, you make your adjustments on where to roll the ball based on the spots since they are two-thirds closer to you. It makes bowling easier and more fun.

In free throw shooting, you start by focusing on the spot on the upper corner tip of the backboard. Next, you move to the regular free throw line and imagine two backboards on each side of the basket running perpendicular from the regular back board. Eventually, you imagine a tube, a funnel, or a slinky extending out from the basket. Once the tube is imagined, then the procedure is similar to SEE-DO.

TUBE — you mentally envision the tube, then you see the ball go through the tube, you hear the cords rip with a swish, which sends emotion through your body and, after experiencing the tingling feeling, you release the ball. Now that you have mentally moved the basket closer, you feel mentally superior and are willing to take a greater risk. As you take a greater risk, you extend the tube. Next, you realize you are not focusing on the rim at all. You are focusing on the opening in the front of the imaginary tube and you are only looking at the rim with your peripheral vision. At this point you realize that what you were taught by your coach — focus on the basket — is a bunch of hogwash which again verifies you are smarter and wiser than your coach.

To utilize the TUBE technique for putting, you place two ball markers six inches from the cup the width of the cup. A ball placed three feet from the cup is now only two feet six inches. You imagine the ball markers making a six-inch tube to the hole. As with basketball free throw shooting, you imagine the ball going through the tube, you hear the plunk, which makes you tingle with excitement, then you stroke the ball. Compared to shooting free throws, you will experience immediate success and you will be tempted to move the ball further away from the hole. Don't. Stay at the three-feet distance and the markers six inches from the hole and concentrate on experiencing the emotion prior to striking the ball. When you feel you are controlling the emotion on a consistent regular basis, begin to move the ball back in six-inch increments. Within a very short period of time you will be knocking down four and five footers. As with the SEE-DO procedure, when you get at the distance it is unreasonable to make the ball go into the hole (making less than 60 percent of the putts), make the hole bigger by drawing a chalk line around the hole. For the average player, you enlarge the hole by two inches when you get beyond seven feet. At 15 to 20 feet, mentally target a hole with a radius within the leather and beyond twenty feet the radius is one club length. You will naturally want to extend the tube by moving the ball markers further from the hole. Moving the markers further back from the hole works for some Level 5s better than others. You are a cognitive person, you think cause and effect, you will figure out what works best for you and, believe me, you will experience success within thirty days with less than thirty minutes of practice a day. Your challenge is to make yourself see the tube, hear the plunk, and feel the tingle **before** striking the ball. You must make your conscious outsmart your subconscious.

The major difference between Level 5 free-throw shooting and putting is you completely control the basketball from the time it is released from your hand to the time it goes through the rim, providing you are not outside or the wind is not blowing. However, imperfections in the green can alter the roll of the ball. So in basketball, when you miss, you flush out the subconscious by consciously saying out loud or to yourself, "That's not like me. That's not the Olympian I know I am." After the flush you refocus. If you are not at the 60 percent accuracy level, move closer. In golf, you must realize you can stroke a ball perfectly and you might miss because of an imperfection in the green. A cleat mark, small bump or indentation can play havoc with a putt. If you strike the ball perfectly and the ball doesn't go in, you flush out the subconscious by consciously reprimanding the green, "That damn spot, it moved my ball." Remember, you are intelligent and you are smart enough to know when it's the green's fault. So, don't consciously try to trick the subconscious into believing you are better than you are when you were perfect to begin with.

Willie Masconi, the great pool shark, taught me this many years ago when he gave a demonstration at the recreational pool hall in Lawrence, Kansas. He came in, chalked up, placed some balls on the table, and began to warm up. As I watched, he was phenomenal. After about five minutes, he was trying a finesse shot in the far right corner, but he kept barely missing it. After the fourth miss, he cursed out loud at the table, jammed his cue stick against the corner of the wall, stomped outside to his car, and returned with a carpenter's level. He placed the level on the table and the pool hall attendants were immediately summoned to put small shims under the corner pocket he kept missing. It might have been all for show, but it impressed me and everyone in the building. I don't remember him missing another shot that day.

Forebrain Dominant, Level 6, Sociocentric
Your strength lies in your sensitivity to others and the environment. Although not particularly competitive, you get a kick out of challenging

yourself. You have abnormal touch and feel. By using the FEEL-SEE-DO process you will learn to fire the front part of your brain and thus control the ball effectively.

In free-throw shooting, you view the ball as an extension of your body. The greater the relationship with the ball, the better the free throw shooter you are. The first mind game you must win is to realize that as you improve your free throw shooting, nobody loses. You are not hurting anyone. This is an individual game that tests your own skill development. This is a way to explore your own mind and its potential.

Once you have determined that free throw shooting is an internal challenge rather than a competitive game, you are ready to begin. The mindset would be the same for learning how to juggle. Before shooting any free throws, you need to heighten your sensitivity to the ball. Rub your hands all over the ball. Rub the ball hard, rub the ball soft. Become super sensitive with the dimples on the ball. Feel the difference between older balls and newer balls. Once you feel intimately in touch with the balls, just go out and shoot free throws for the fun of it. Don't count how many you make or don't make, just stop shooting when it is no longer fun. When you catch yourself shooting just to be shooting, stop. When your brain fires in the front, it is enjoyable. The second it is no longer enjoyable, the brain begins to fire hemispherically. You want the brain to continue to fire in the front with hypersensitivity and joy. After shooting free throws for the fun of it, go listen to music. Listen to various types of music. Select six different pieces of music that move you or make you feel different. Now play the music as you shoot free throws for fun. Again, don't count how many shots you make or don't make. You are attempting to enhance your feeling.

Within a couple of enjoyable free-throw sessions, you will select a piece of music that causes an emotional reaction within you. This emotional reaction will be deep within your chest and will enhance your awareness to the ball and the environment. Now play the music while you shoot and there will be times you get in sync with the music. The feeling you get while you are in sync helps you glide the ball through the hole. This feeling is uncanny and words won't adequately describe what is going on, but you will know it and sense it when it happens. Your goal is to increase the length of time (or number of consecutive shots) you are in sync. While in sync, your sensitivity and awareness are so intact you can't miss. When you are out of sync you lose all feeling and you become awkward and out of touch. As the length of time in sync increases, begin to learn how to feel in sync without music. Within a few days you will no longer need the music because you will be able to mentally hear the beat, the rhythm, the tone, and the volume. As you mentally hear the music, you must begin to mentally feel in sync. Now keep track of the number of shots you make in a row.

FEEL — mentally hear the music, feel the dimples, feel in sync, SEE the ball mentally go through the hoop, hear the ball rip the cords, feel the tingle, then DO — release the ball. Record consecutive successful shots made, not percentages. As the number of consecutive successful shots increases, your awareness will greatly increase to the point you will become very excited and anxious each time before you shoot. You are controlling the firing in the front part of your brain. At this point, begin to record percentages of shots made. When you miss, flush your mind, as in free-throw shooting, Levels 4 and 5.

Forebrain free-throw shooters take longer to experience success, but once you get in sync and after you learn to control the firing of your brain through the FEEL-SEE-DO process, you will master free throw shooting and become Olympian. You have the natural mental makeup to be a 90 percent plus free-throw shooter within 30 days of practice. You begin counting the 30 days when you no longer need the music.

As a putter, you get intimately familiar with the putter. Feel the grip as well as the head. Test the sweet spot on the putter by gently holding the putter high in the air with one hand and with the other take a metal pointed object like a knife blade or car key and poke it at different places along the face of the putter. You will feel the putter twist and turn in your outstretched hand when you strike the putter head outside the sweet spot. When you hit the sweet spot, the putter will feel solid and it won't twist and turn in your hand. Before putting any balls to a hole, you must first be able to strike the ball on the sweet spot every time. Hitting the ball on the sweet spot will send a feeling of confidence up through your hands and into your body. However, you want hitting the ball on the sweet spot to transfer to your subconscious. To get this feeling of successfully hitting the ball on the sweet spot, you merely tap the ball around the green, focusing on hitting the ball on the sweet spot. Do not try to knock the ball into a hole. Just tap the ball on the sweet spot. Being a Level 6, you will have no trouble finding the sweet spot and you are so sensitive you will know immediately when you hit the ball on the sweet spot. Furthermore, you will get the knack of hitting the ball on the sweet spot within 10 to 15 minutes of concentrated practice.

As you get better and you feel what it is like to hit the ball on the sweet spot, begin to hit the ball harder until you are hitting it 20 to 30 feet. Now begin to lag the ball to a ten foot line but, before striking the ball, mentally FEEL what it is like, SEE the ball come close to the lag line, experience the tingle, then DO — strike the ball. As you gain confidence, now place six balls in a circle three feet from the hole. As you putt, pile the balls up into the hole until it overflows. As the cup fills up and as it begins to overflow, you will become more excited and you can't wait to do it again. At this point you are controlling the subconscious.

FEEL-SEE-DO. FEEL the sweet spot, SEE the ball go into the hole, hear it plunk to the bottom of the cup, feel the tingle, and DO — stroke one ball. Repeat the process until all six balls are putted. As you practice, always use six balls and always put them in a circle around the cup. As you improve, increase the distance in six inch increments. Most Level 6 golfers don't need music to help them; however, if you feel it might help, use a Walkman rather than a Boom box.

As with free throw shooting, it will take you a little longer to get started, but your putting will become masterful within less than 30 days from the time you start putting six balls around the cup. You have the mental makeup to be a masterful putter because the skill of putting is mostly feel and touch. Let the conscious tell the subconscious what to do through the FEEL-SEE-DO process. Putting is feel and touch AND 99 PER-CENT MENTAL.

Rearbrain Dominant, Level 7, Cognitive

Your strength lies in your internal motivation, healthy sense of balance, and joy of capturing the moment. When you get focused on a singular issue, you "will" it to happen. You "will" it to happen by getting into the flow or zone. Mihaly Csikszentmihalyi has helped us understand the flow through his ideas about "the psychology of optimal experience." The flow is a state of mind in which people get so involved that nothing else matters. The experience is so joyful that they will continue in the activity over and over again even at great effort and/or sacrifice. When in the flow it is effortless, like being carried by a current. The goals are crystal clear and the feedback is constant and constructive. In free throw shooting, you know whether the ball goes in the hole or out, in singing you hear yourself hitting the right notes or not. Great concentration is experienced by sensing a balance between what you can do with what to do. While experiencing the flow the activity is absorbing, interesting and fun. A mountain climber needs a goal of getting to the top. But the goal of getting to the top is nothing more than an excuse to climb. If there is no joy in climbing, then it is a wasted activity. The process is more important than the goal, although it is important to attain the goal. While in the flow, you transcend time and space; you get so caught up in the activity you lose track of time and you forget where you are; yet you are aware of every single thing about you. The key to controlling the firing of the rear part of the brain is to consciously slip into the zone and let the subconscious take over. By using the BIRDMAN process, you will learn how to slip into the zone.

The BIRDMAN process was developed after watching Larry Bird rapidly shoot three-point shots during the annual three-point shot contest. Each year he would appear to get into a zone and experience such joy, one might identify it as ecstasy. He was focused, his shooting was effortless, he had exceptional concentration, and the balls kept going through the basket. As one watched more closely, it was noticed he would shoot one ball, but before it reached the basket, he would be releasing another ball as the previous ball just reached the rim. Most of the time, as he shot balls moving around the three-point arc, two balls were always in the air. Upon closer observation, it appeared he didn't look at the basket but was focused about four to five feet from his extended shooting hand, as if he had a point or spot for the ball to cross. The point or spot was akin to the sight at the end of a barrel on a rifle, except the sight and the barrel were both imaginary. Apparently he had a sense of where he was in relationship to the basket and caught the basket in his peripheral vision while focusing on the imaginary sight four to five feet from his extended shooting hand.

Using the BIRDMAN process for shooting free throws, we extend the tube, slinky, out from our extended shooting hand rather than from the basket, as is done in the Level 5, TUBE process. To teach yourself this process, extend your shooting hand out toward the basket, pointing to the site you want the ball to go over about four to five feet from your pointed finger while holding the ball in your nonshooting hand, the guiding hand, so-to-speak. Next, focus on the site, see the ball pass over the site, then actually shoot the ball. You will miss a lot of shots in the beginning, but once you make a shot or two, a feeling of ecstasy will fall over you. Remember, never focus directly on the basket, always see the basket using your peripheral vision. It is difficult to explain, but for some reason you experience a mini-high as the ball rips the cords. Since you are not looking directly at the basket, it is almost magic. After experiencing this feeling, you will realize why players like Bird and Jordan would practice hours on end, to the point of exhaustion — this process is actually addictive. Now that you have sensed the mini-high, your challenge is to control the emotion rather than letting the swishing of the ball going through the net trigger the high. You do this by: focus on the site, see the ball pass over the site, **feel the sensation of the high**, release the ball. As a Level 7, when you miss you don't have to flush the missed shot or the feeling of missing the shot out of your mind. You just shoot another shot because while in the zone you are always on an emotional high all the time, making constant adjustments. You are in the zone, your brain is firing in the rear, and the brain will subconsciously keep correcting the flight of the ball as you "will" it to happen.

To enhance this feeling, shoot several balls rapidly from the free-throw line and establish a rhythm. A rhythm will intensify the flow. This becomes even greater as you choose basketballs with different textures. To get different textures, get balls from different manufacturers, use some old balls, some new, and use some leather balls and some rubber. As a Level 7, getting in the flow will not be a new experience for you, but what will be new is now you know how to control getting into the flow as compared to it just happening on occasion. In other words, you will be able to get in the flow on demand. You cause the flow to happen rather than just experience the flow out of doing an activity.

As a putter, to use the BIRDMAN process you imagine the sight on the barrel to be six to ten inches from the ball rather than from the hole. As a Level 7, you will not need to use ball markers to guide you. You will intuitively see the sight. Getting into the flow in golf is easier while putting than while shooting free throws in basketball because you are always focusing on the golf ball before you strike it and not on the cup. It is more natural to focus on the golf ball, while in basketball it is more natural to focus on the rim.

One individual who was learning the **PeopleWise® Motivation** techniques and who had played both basketball and golf at the college level burst out, "Ah-hah. I got it now. I used to get much more excited when I sank a putt than when I swished a basket. It is all so simple. Now, when I make a basket using my peripheral vision to see the rim, the mini-high I get is equal to the mini-high I experience when I sink a putt. The key is in Level 7 thinking. It is magical."

Another difference between basketball and golf is, to get in the zone in golf you don't want rhythm. The zone in golf is all mental, in basketball it is more holistic — mind, body, kinesthetic. The game of golf lends itself to more level 7 stuff. Most golfers experience the zone from time to time. When you are in the zone, you cause things to happen, you "will" it, you can't miss. At other times you are completely out of it. As a Level 7, you can enhance the feeling of ecstasy and increase your control of the zone by never putting the ball from the same distance. The reason you change distances every time is because when you play golf for real you don't have a practice shot first to get the feel and direction of the green. The feel and direction must be generated mentally. In the zone you don't need practice shots, you mentally have a sense of everything. As a Level 7, on the practice green, every time you putt the ball the same distance from the hole you are consciously telling the subconscious you need to hit a practice ball first to get the feeling and direction before you hit for real. When you play for real and you can't test the green with a trial putt you have consciously telegraphed to the subconscious you can't do it. In other words, you think when you putt balls the same distance from the hole you are gaining confidence, the truth is with Level 7s you are telling your subconscious you need a crutch. Your confidence is lowered in direct proportion to the number of putts you roll the same distance from the hole. Let's say you are five feet from the hole and in practice you hit ten balls from the same exact spot. You miss the first two, make one, miss three, and make the last four.

You leave the green satisfied and falsely confident. Now you play for real and you end up on the same green in the same exact spot. I ask you, how confident are you now? On the practice green you have successfully knocked the ball in the hole half the time. Now, for real, do you think you have a 50% chance of making it? Of course not. Your subconscious has taken control and is telegraphing to you loud and clear, you are no good without a couple of practice rolls; there is no way you can get the ball in the hole the first time. During practice you have programmed your mind for failure.

In addition to not putting the same distance from the cup, you can enhance your feeling of ecstasy and increase your control of getting in the zone by never putting with the same putter twice. Take three or four putters to the practice green with you. Alternate putters every shot and never putt the ball from the same distance twice. As you use the BIRD-MAN process, you will consciously telegraph to your subconscious that you are more important than the putter. You can "will" the ball in the hole. While in the zone, you cause the future through post-living.

PeopleWise® Motivation is a theory. It is not to be confused with the truth. However, the PeopleWise® Motivation theory provides us with four distinct and different processes to use to improve our own skill development. The processes are unambiguous and provide methods to try that are clear, concise, and doable. Each of the four processes are grounded in an understandable philosophy. Each process can be tested to determine its worth.

To determine the effectiveness of the theory of **PeopleWise® Motivation** you simply select a skill you want to improve that can be counted and/or measured. You first execute the skill as best you can and record the percent of successes. Keep in mind, to adequately assess **PeopleWise® Motivation**, your present skill level must be at the 60 percent accuracy level or above in order to properly control the firing of the brain. If it is below 60 percent, adjust the goal, skill, process in such a way that you attain 60 percent success. As you record the successes of your selected skill, you eventually will reach a leveling off or plateau. The plateau's average is what you want to beat. This will be your baseline from which to measure the power of **PeopleWise® Motivation**. Next, you pick a method, Level 4, 5, 6 or 7, that you think will work for you.

If you are unsure of what Level to start with, read the next chapter, Chapter 16, Assessing the Activation of Your Own Brain. Once you select a method, begin to execute the process as previously prescribed. Execute the selected process for thirty days, recording the percentage of successes each day. This is your treatment — Treatment A. After thirty days, average the percentages of your treatment and compare it with the average of your plateau baseline. If the difference is a lot greater, five percentage points or higher, then **PeopleWise® Motivation** is working for you. If it is not at least five percentage points higher, you might want to select another Level. This will be Treatment B. Record successful percentages each day for thirty days, then average the percentages from Treatment B and determine how it faired with your baseline. The beauty of **PeopleWise® Motivation** is you can play around with it various ways and lengths of time to determine what works and what doesn't. If it doesn't work, just sell your book in the next garage sale and hopefully it will work for the next person. Figure 15-1 shows a format you might want to try for graphing and keeping track of your percentages.

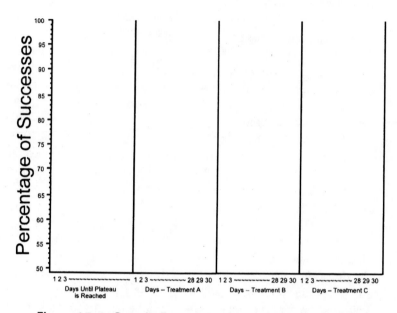

Figure 15-1. Sample Format for Recording and Graphing Percentages of Successes to Determine the Power of PeopleWise® Motivation

CHAPTER SIXTEEN

ASSESSING THE ACTIVATION OF YOUR OWN BRAIN

ust exactly what is **PeopleWise® Motivation**? **PeopleWise® Motivation** is a theory on the connection between how people behave with the activation of the brain. It is really a theory of theories. **PeopleWise® Motivation** begins with the personal development field of visual imagery and mental rehearsal, and builds on the base of Dr. Clare Grave's Levels of Psychological Existence, which contends the brain and the environment interact with one another and form a predictable ascending staircase of steps with identifiable Levels, and finally takes information related to brain activation which indicates that as an individual becomes focused, the firing of the brain becomes more localized.

PeopleWise® Motivation gives us some ideas on how to motivate ourselves, how to motivate others, and how to improve our own skill development by mastering the control of our own brain activation. Many paper/pencil instruments have been developed to identify various personality traits. The following, **PeopleWise® Self-Assessment System**, identifies ways and means that individuals can use to understand their preferred Level of functioning, where an individual's brain is most likely to activate, and subsequently, how an individual can go ahead improving skill development by controlling one's concentration, focus, and confidence.

The **PeopleWise®** Self-Assessment System produces a graphic depiction of where the brain may have a tendency to activate. Once the preferred brain location and activation intensity are determined, then a suggestion can be made regarding the Level of functioning and how an individual may go about mentally improving one's own skill development. The **PeopleWise®** Self-Assessment System is provided to only give a ballpark idea of where an individual is functioning.

PEOPLEWISE® SELF–ASSESSMENT SYSTEM

Following each of the 21 statements below are four possible choices. Select the sentence, phrase, or word that describes you best or that you prefer most. Place an X in the appropriate box. If more than one choice appeals to you, force yourself to just pick one that appeals to you and move on. Keep in mind, this is not a test. There are no right or wrong answers. You can't pass or fail. The purpose of the instrument is to give you a ball park reading regarding your Level of functioning and where and at what intensity your brain is firing.

Put an x in the box of your choice. ONLY ONE X FOR EACH STATEMENT.

1. I FEEL IT IS IMPORTANT TO:

☐ A. Be steady and secure
☐ B. Be seen by others as important and respected
☐ C. Have many fine friends and acquaintances
☐ D. Develop and realize my full potential

2. THIS I BELIEVE ABOUT FRIENDSHIP:

☐ A. It is a lasting and permanent relationship
☐ B. It is a give and take process
☐ C. Without friends life is nothing
☐ D. Some people need friends, some people don't

3. THE WORD THAT DESCRIBES ME BEST IS:

☐ A. Reliable
☐ B. Competitive
☐ C. Reflective
☐ D. Transcending

4. I ENJOY SITUATIONS WHICH PROVIDE AN OPPORTUNITY FOR ME TO:

- ☐ A. Increase my prestige and receive well-deserved attention
- ☐ B. Develop plans and programs for my future
- ☐ C. Meet new people and make new friends
- ☐ D. Utilize talents and capabilities I don't often use

5. THIS I BELIEVE ABOUT THE AMERICAN WAY OF LIFE:

- ☐ A. McDonald's is taking over
- ☐ B. Competition has brought about highest standards of living ever achieved in history
- ☐ C. Church, Mom, apple pie, best there is
- ☐ D. Confused society with misplaced values

6. THE WORD THAT DESCRIBES ME BEST IS:

- ☐ A. Contextual
- ☐ B. Cordial
- ☐ C. Driven
- ☐ D. Consistent

7. I TEND TO PLACE THE GREATEST EMPHASIS ON:

- ☐ A. Developing self-confidence, pride, and influence over others
- ☐ B. The achievement of personal goals and objectives
- ☐ C. Building a secure life for myself and others who may be dependent on me
- ☐ D. Being with and enjoying the company of my friends

8. THIS I BELIEVE ABOUT SIN:

- ☐ A. There are no levels of sin – wrong is wrong
- ☐ B. Sin is everywhere
- ☐ C. No such thing – dreamed up to scare people
- ☐ D. Different people consider different things sin

9. THE WORD THAT DESCRIBES ME BEST IS:

☐ A. Entrepreneurial
☐ B. Dependable
☐ C. Childlike (not child-ish)
☐ D. Altruistic

10. FROM TIME TO TIME I THINK ABOUT:

☐ A. My safety and security
☐ B. Increasing my competence
☐ C. Improving myself so that I could do even more worthwhile and challenging things
☐ D. Getting to know people, pleasing them, and maintaining their friendship

11. THIS I BELIEVE ABOUT MARRIAGE:

☐ A. A state of mind, not a piece of paper
☐ B. A way to insure that both partners try harder to stay together
☐ C. Sacred union of two people who love each other and should be faithful to one another
☐ D. Good for some, bad for others

12. THE WORD THAT DESCRIBES ME BEST IS:

☐ A. Change-oriented
☐ B. Inventive
☐ C. Orthodox
☐ D. Amiable

13. I TEND TO LOOK FOR:

☐ A. Friendly people who support one another
☐ B. Freedom and an opportunity to grow as much as I can
☐ C. Recognition for outstanding performance
☐ D. Consistency, stability, and security

14. THIS I BELIEVE ABOUT RELIGION:

- ☐ A. It is necessary for living a full and meaningful life
- ☐ B. It is interesting and important to many people
- ☐ C. People generally need someone or something to believe in
- ☐ D. Religion is becoming too commercial

15. THE WORD THAT DESCRIBES ME BEST IS:

- ☐ A. People-oriented
- ☐ B. Industrious
- ☐ C. Totality
- ☐ D. Persistent

16. I WOULD BECOME DISCOURAGED IF:

- ☐ A. Things became mundane and I found myself doing the same things over and over again
- ☐ B. The overall conditions became unstable and depressed
- ☐ C. I started to be taken for granted and was by-passed on some promotional opportunities
- ☐ D. I ended up doing work by myself with very little opportunity to see or work with others

17. THIS I BELIEVE ABOUT OTHER PEOPLE:

- ☐ A. People are basically no good, but I love them anyway
- ☐ B. People make me feel secure
- ☐ C. People, as I see them, are beautiful, if only the world could be beautiful with all those people
- ☐ D. People are the most unique set of organisms in the world

18. THE WORD THAT DESCRIBES ME BEST IS:

- ☐ A. Companionable
- ☐ B. Loyal
- ☐ C. Adventurous
- ☐ D. Inner-directed

19. WHAT IS VERY IMPORTANT TO ME IS:

- ☐ A. Being part of a top-notch group with good fellowship
- ☐ B. Knowing that I am one of "the best" and being respected for it
- ☐ C. Being required to stretch a little, tackle a difficult task, and see the results
- ☐ D. Clear-cut ground rules, and reasonable protection

20. THIS I BELIEVE ABOUT RULES:

- ☐ A. Too much emphasis on them
- ☐ B. Useful if reasonable
- ☐ C. I can take them or leave them, but I try to obey most of the important rules
- ☐ D. Are made to be obeyed

21. THE WORD THAT DESCRIBES ME BEST IS:

- ☐ A. Sensing
- ☐ B. Conventional
- ☐ C. Fearless
- ☐ D. Persuasive

ANALYSIS FOR PEOPLEWISE® SELF-ASSESSMENT SYSTEM

INSTRUCTIONS: Place your choices with an X alongside the alternatives (A, B, C, or D) in the space below. Work across the sheet for each of the twenty-one statements. Remember, you will have three blanks for each statement. Then add the X's in each column to obtain your Totals.

1A _____	1B _____	1C _____	1D _____
2A _____	2B _____	2C _____	2D _____
3A _____	3B _____	3C _____	3D _____
4B _____	4A _____	4C _____	4D _____
5C _____	5B _____	5D _____	5A _____
6D _____	6C _____	6B _____	6A _____
7C _____	7A _____	7D _____	7B _____
8A _____	8B _____	8C _____	8D _____
9B _____	9A _____	9D _____	9C _____
10A _____	10B _____	10D _____	10C _____
11C _____	11B _____	11A _____	11D _____
12C _____	12A _____	12D _____	12B _____
13D _____	13C _____	13A _____	13B _____
14A _____	14C _____	14D _____	14B _____
15D _____	15B _____	15A _____	15C _____
16B _____	16C _____	16D _____	16A _____
17B _____	17D _____	17C _____	17A _____
18B _____	18C _____	18A _____	18D _____
19D _____	19B _____	19A _____	19C _____
20D _____	20B _____	20A _____	20C _____
21B _____	21D _____	21A _____	21C _____

TOTAL	☐	☐	☐	☐
LEVEL	4	5	6	7
LOCATION	LEFT	RIGHT	FRONT	REAR

To chart your brain activation and intensity, take your totals from the analysis (previous page) and block in (use pencil or pen) the number of cells for each level in the Brain Activation Graphic (Figure 16-2). For clarity, block in the cells as indicated by the numbers within the cells. For example, TOTAL (13) LEVEL 4 LEFT, (3) LEVEL 5 RIGHT, (4) LEVEL 6 FRONT, (1) LEVEL 7 REAR (See Figure 16-1 below). This person is predominately functioning at Level 4 and firing in the left hemisphere.

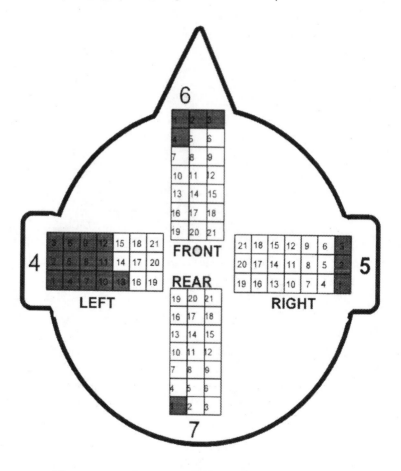

Figure 16-1: Example of Brain Activation Graphic
(13 LEVEL 4 LEFT, 3 LEVEL 5 RIGHT, 4 LEVEL 6 FRONT, 1 LEVEL 7 REAR)

PeopleWise® Self-Assessment System
Brain Activation Graphic

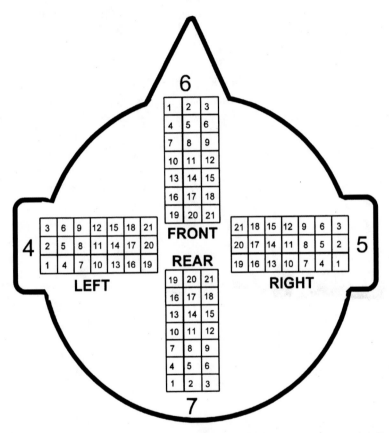

Figure 16-2: Brain Activation Graphic, block in the number of cells
for each level.
Use your totals from the Analysis for PeopleWise® Self-Assessment
Systems page 181.

For a ballpark interpretation of your results, study your completed Brain Activation Graphic. The following section, **PeopleWise®** Pattern Descriptions, contains the basic Levels. If the bulk of your scores fall in a particular Level or area, turn to an explanation of that Level. If you are a combination of Levels, with no clear apparent pattern, turn to the Blends. The basic patterns included are:

LEVELS: 4, 5, 6, 7

BLENDS: 4-5, 5-6, 4-6

For persons whose scores fall outside these basic patterns, the **PeopleWise® Profile System** is available. The **PeopleWise® Profile System** is more sophisticated and has more options. For information on the PeopleWise® Profile System, call or write for a free brochure and catalog:

Management & Motivation, Inc.
P.O. Box 215
University, MS 38677
(662) 234-8846
mm@watervalley.net
FAX #: (662) 281-8780

PEOPLEWISE® PATTERN
DESCRIPTIONS

PEOPLEWISE® PATTERN DESCRIPTIONS

LEVEL 4, ABSOLUTIST

Characteristics

You are driven by principle. You have high standards and high expectations for yourself and others. You will sacrifice for those things you believe are important. You work hard and some may believe you work too hard. If you agree to do it, you do it. You have a tenacity that you believe is focused while others may see you as dogged. You are steady and can be counted on. You don't seek recognition but expect to be treated fair. You are undemonstrative, but if pushed, can show anger or at least hold your ground and be firm. You are sensitive to manipulation and may occasionally wonder what people are up to or what they want. You want to know what is expected of you, how you will be evaluated, what the goals are, and what the time lines are. You work best in a predictable environment and you will shoulder more than your share without complaint. When the going gets tough, the tough get going. You are not hesitant to put your shoulder to the wheel or put your nose to the grindstone. You are a meat and potatoes type of no-frills person. You can put off until tomorrow and save for a rainy day.

Self Motivation

Your brain activates predominately in the left hemisphere. Your skill improves under a regimen or system that moves from Step 1, to Step 2, to Step 3, etc. You are good at following guidelines and you feel comfortable with principles that help with improved skill development. You can benefit from watching an expert that you respect and admire. Your skill improves by periodically reminding yourself to go back to the basics. Review your stance, head placement and position of arms — whatever is appropriate for the skill you are mastering. The object is to get your complex body to do the same movement, time and time again. In your case, practice does make perfect, providing you stick to the basics. Don't over-think and don't over-analyze your movement. Just repeat your movement exactly as it should be done again and again and again. See yourself doing it right. Visualize yourself doing it exactly as it is to be done. Become mentally tough. Work your mind as hard as you work your body. You can benefit from some muscle memory training that teaches you how to perfect your movement through modeling a perfect motion. One of the most effective ways to utilize muscle memory training is to study a video or compact disk of a professional executing the desired skill and then you physically repeating the movement over and over. Your skill improvement lies in repetition of doing it right again and again and again and again.

Strengths

Things done right; reliable; high standards; self discipline; good follow through/follow up

Weaknesses

Sometimes over-opinionated; suspicious; worrisome; at times over does it; resistant to change

Improvement

Be more flexible; share with others more; become more visionary; try out new things; take calculated risks

PEOPLEWISE® PATTERN DESCRIPTIONS

LEVEL 5, MATERIALIST

Characteristics

You are competitive. You have high energy. You like to win and you challenge yourself. You have an internal desire that pushes you to exceed. You have unusual bursts of energy. You don't need much sleep. You enjoy life and consider yourself zestful. You express yourself openly and some consider you animated or possibly outspoken. You are spirited and very active. You like to do a variety of things and are spontaneous. You search for new and different ways to do things. You like change. Although you can set goals, you find oftentimes you exceed your expectations and end up in places and situations you hadn't planned for. You like yourself and are confident. You will take a calculated risk and you learn from your mistakes. You don't look back. You are a no-nonsense person and want to get on with it. You don't like to waste time, yet you enjoy time. You work hard but, more importantly, you work smart. You like to think things out and occasionally scribble random isolated ideas down on paper. When the going gets tough, you get competitive. You stand tall and walk with authority. You project enthusiasm. You plan for tomorrow but believe tomorrow is now.

Self Motivation

Your brain activates predominately in the right hemisphere. Your skill improves with study, calculation, and analysis. For you, practice does not make perfect. For you, perfect practice makes perfect. Your time is valuable, therefore, your practice must be focused and intense. You are a cause-and-effect person. You believe you can cause things to happen. You like to act on the environment. The important thing is not doing it exactly right, the important thing is doing it with maximum effort and, of course, accomplishing the goal. For you, desire is more important than basics. The body is complex and the job is to achieve, even when your body is out of sync. You do this by mind over matter, visualizing what you want to accomplish, where the ball is to go, the end result. This type of visualization will help you achieve and excel. You can't over-analyze or over-think. You are a cognitive being. Going back to basics is a waste of time for you and is boring. Do not try to visualize your movement — you must project out and visualize what is to happen rather than how it is to be done. You can greatly benefit from practicing visual imagery and mental rehearsal. Once you catch onto how to use visual imagery and mental rehearsal, your skill level will take a quantum-leap forward.

Strengths

Focus; high energy; calculated risks; attainment of goals; achievement

Weaknesses

Impulsive; erratic; impatient; outspoken; at times, too self-congratulatory

Improvement

Listen more; slow down; schedule time for self; write to your mother; take time to smell the roses

PEOPLEWISE® PATTERN DESCRIPTIONS

LEVEL 6, SOCIOCENTRIC

Characteristics

You are a people person. You have a sensitivity that is exceptional. You are an excellent listener and people enjoy being in your presence. You don't just listen, you get involved in the situation and others can sense you are engaged with them. Your body language and eye contact express honesty, sensitivity, concern, and deep feeling. You are a giver, an unconditional giver, that expects nothing in return. However, if someone pays you back for the kindnesses you unselfishly bestowed, you will humbly, almost embarrassingly, accept, but deep down you wish they had not reciprocated. You have a hypersensitivity to how people feel — happy/sad, excited/depressed, joyful/angry, and apathetic/concerned ... Regardless of the situation, you remain optimistic, positive, and most importantly, hopeful. You are not goal-driven, you are purpose-driven. You take time to smell the roses. When the going gets tough, the tough get sensitive. You are not so much interested in the past or the future, but focus on the present — what is happening to us now, what we are feeling, what is really going on between us at this moment in time. Spontaneity, creativity, and expression of self are key to your very being.

Self Motivation

Your brain activates predominately in the front. Your skill improves when you feel the process or you get into your rhythm. One of the difficulties regarding skill improvement is directly related to you not wanting to beat another person or win at the expense of the other person losing. Therefore, you are not competitively motivated to improve. You are not driven to win. What is important to you is, did we have fun, did we do our best, did we work as a team, and did we learn. One way to help you improve a skill is to measure your improvement against yourself. As you become more skilled, you gain an appreciation for yourself, not because you can beat anyone, but because you see yourself getting better. Sometimes you may be wise to transfer your skill development to the arts as opposed to sports. If you want to improve a sports skill, once you have mastered the basics, you will find you are a natural for studying psycho cybernetics. This basic type of visual imaging and mental rehearsal benefits you because it relies on feeling the success **before** it happens. You feel the success by visualizing the outcome of the skill before execution. Once you feel the thrill by mentally seeing the outcome, you are in a position to increase your concentration, focus, and confidence. It is unlikely your skill will improve with a step-by-step regimented program or an intense study of the skill through calculation and analysis. For you, practice doesn't make perfect nor does perfect practice make perfect. For you, mentally practicing, visualizing, feeling the rhythm is as important as actually physically practicing once you have mastered the basics. Anything you can do to heighten the feeling of success will enhance your skill.

Strengths

Sensitivity; purposeful intentions; caring; sharing; team player

Weaknesses

Can't say no; others control time; appear to lack direction; will settle for less; indecisive at times

Improvement

Set personal goals; learn to tactfully say no; become proactive; spend time with people not like you; master a physical skill

PEOPLEWISE® PATTERN DESCRIPTIONS

LEVEL 7, COGNITIVE

Characteristics

You hold yourself in high esteem and see yourself as principle-centered, internally motivated, and destined to make things happen that contribute to the greater good. You are intrigued with existence itself and enjoy living life to its fullest. You are complex and live multiple lives. You need little sleep and your mind is always running at full speed. You never get depressed, but sometimes you get confused, especially when you witness injustices. However, you seek clarity through meditation and/or solitude and you are back on track before you know it. You enjoy ambiguity, variety, differences, and occasionally, chaos. You view the world contextually, thus, you can handle, value and appreciate extreme differences in opinions and life styles. You have conquered fear. You have either had a brush with death or intimately know of someone that has. You have no fear of boss, survival, social acceptance, political pressure, economic strife, or death. You are autonomous, inner-directed, and are cognizantly complex. You work on many things at once, yet you are focused on each multi-task. On occasion, you can get so focused on a singular issue you actually "will" it to happen. You think and behave so differently from the masses that your close friends admire you and have extreme high regard for you. Your enemies fear you and are confused by your activities. Many outsiders see you as unique, odd, different and/or possibly crazy. The world is a better place because of you. You are not interested in the past, present or future. You are interested in process. While others ponder if there is life after death, you wonder if there is life after birth.

Self Motivation

Your brain activates predominately in the rear. When you want, your skill level may become Olympian; however, since you are more interested in processes and experiences than you are in outcomes, you may excel in spurts, just to see if you can do it. You love to test limits and you like to do things out of the ordinary: balloon, mountain climb, juggle, etc. You can master the basics of most any skill in much less time than most people and you understand the value of focus, concentration and confidence. True skill excellence will be achieved by trying it in an entirely different way than it has been done before. If you select a skill that intrigues you and you stay with it for a significant period of time, you will excel. How can you get yourself to stay with something for a significant period of time? No one knows, but experience and observation suggest that the skill must fascinate you to the point you will test the existing limits, time and time again. The best advice is to look for answers outside the skill itself, but, of course, you already know that.

Strengths

Intensity; focus; self-assurance; joy; contribute to the greater good

Weaknesses

Unwillingness to please; enjoys chaos and, at times, causes chaos; disruptive; too frank; too self-righteous

Improvement

Teach others; keep records on personal insights; say I'm sorry and please; be kind to those close to you; cheer down

PEOPLEWISE® PATTERN DESCRIPTIONS

LEVEL 4-5, ABSOLUTIST-MATERIALIST BLEND

Characteristics

You are the best of two worlds: solid work ethic coupled with the right amount of drive and desire. You are competitive, yet you play by the rules. Sportsmanship is important to you. You lead by your actions and deeds. People see you as healthy and purposeful. People admire your level-headedness. You plan things out and have the energy to carry out your plan. Sometimes you get caught in a dilemma; you want things done right, yet you want things done in a timely manner. Pushed to an extreme, you may, on occasion, want things done perfect and you want things done immediately. These opposing drives place you in a predicament that forces excellence — top quality in breakneck speed. This dual drive, when mastered, places you head and shoulders above your peers and competitors. However, this dual drive, when unmastered, may occasionally lead to indecision, confusion, and possibly chaos. When you are unsure you are best advised to slow down and make your decision based on your principles and standards. When in doubt, think things out. You might get some insights into yourself by studying LEVEL 4, ABSOLUTIST and LEVEL 5, MATERIALIST. Keep in mind you are a combination of both. You are able to take the best of both. One does not compromise the other.

Self Motivation

Your brain activates in both the right and left hemispheres. Skill improvement is best when you follow a two-phase process. First, you master the basics. This is done by focusing on proper positioning of your body and execution of the ideal, traditional muscle movement, i.e., proper stance and proper body movement. Once you master the basics without having to think, you move to the second phase, which is all mental. Here you focus on training your brain to visualize the outcome. Before execution, you first see in your "mind's eye" exactly the perfect outcome, then you must feel what it is like to succeed. This feeling of success or accomplishment gives you confidence. Confidence is knowing you are going to be successful before execution. After you feel the success, you actually begin execution of your skill movement. People who become very good at a skill develop an Olympian focus. For you, first work the left side of the brain, mastering the basics, then activate the right side of the brain through visualizing the outcome. To get a better grasp of the procedure, read and master the Self Motivation section for LEVEL 4, ABSOLUTIST, then proceed to LEVEL 5, MATERIALIST. You are going to move from practice makes perfect to perfect practice makes perfect.

Strengths

Self discipline; high energy; achievement; good follow through

Weaknesses

At times overdoes it; impulsive; sometimes over-opinionated; impatient

Improvement

Become more visionary; listen more; try out new things; slow down

PEOPLEWISE® PATTERN DESCRIPTIONS

LEVEL 5-6, MATERIALIST-SOCIOCENTRIC BLEND

Characteristics

You are the best of two worlds: healthy drive and desire, coupled with the right amount of sensitivity. You get the job done with heart. Accomplishment is important as are people's opinions and feelings. You are a great coach. You have a knack for getting things done. You can lead by example or you can convince people to do things by cheering them on from the sidelines. Winning is important, but never more important than learning. You are into doing while, at the same time, being. You have a strong desire to assist people in their development, growth, and maturation while they are accomplishing a task or experiencing victory. You don't have much of a dilemma in your life because you have figured out winning is only as important as what is accomplished through winning. For you, winning is not a goal, winning is a process. You might get some insights into yourself by studying LEVEL 5, MATERIALIST and LEVEL 6, SOCIOCENTRIC. Keep in mind, you are a combination of both. You are able to take the best of both. One does not compromise the other.

Self Motivation

Your brain activates in both the right and front. Skill improvement is developing the "will" to make it happen. This is difficult because you have a tendency to want to run before you walk. You like to experiment and try things out. You are constantly questioning and experimenting. You are best advised to play around with your skill development. Read, study, get video training tapes, and study different techniques and philosophies. Once you decide on the philosophy and technique you are going to use, begin to spend the majority of your time preparing for the mental part. Your brain activates on the right side, which is excellent for studying cause and effect. You have excellent analytical skills. You use the right side of the brain to determine which philosophy or technique is best for you. After the decision is made on what is best for you, you begin to activate the front part of the brain to get a feeling for what it is like to execute perfectly. By combining the right and front parts of the brain you develop a "will" for perfection. This "will" for perfection can give you a competitive edge; however, this "will" can only be achieved through rigorous mental training. Without disciplined, rigorous training you have a tendency to see the activity for what it is, just a game. At this point your interest turns to enjoying the activity as opposed to mastering the skill. You use the game to experience life or to learn about yourself. True mastery comes from disciplined mental training, but it isn't easy. Read the motivation section on LEVEL 6, SOCIOCENTRIC and LEVEL 5, MATERIAL-IST. This may give you an insight into your complex self.

Strengths

High energy; sensitive, purposeful intentions; achievement

Weaknesses

Will settle for less; impulsive; impatient; resistant to trivia or basics

Improvement

Be proactive; study and listen more; master a physical skill; slow down

PEOPLEWISE® PATTERN DESCRIPTIONS

LEVEL 4-6, ABSOLUTIST-SOCIOCENTRIC BLEND

Characteristics

You are the best of two worlds: solid work ethic coupled with the right amount of sensitivity. You value standards, policies and rules, yet you have a true feeling for people and how procedures effect people. You do things right and, at the same time, you do the right things. People admire your healthiness. As you plan things out you constantly weigh how people will react yet, at the same time, you understand that for the organization to survive, things must move forward in a timely fashion. You are able to get things accomplished through people but, if necessary, you can roll your sleeves up and do it yourself. Sometimes you get caught in a dilemma — you want things done right, yet you want people to like what they do. Because you are psychologically very healthy, these opposing drives of getting things done with happy, contented people brings out the best in everyone. However, on occasion, these opposing drives may cause you to hesitate or delay an action. When you are unsure, you are best advised to consider the greater good or the contribution to the whole because healthy individuals are adaptable and realize things can't always go their way. As long as the decision is based on what is best for the greater good or whole, everything else will fall in place. You might get some insights into yourself by studying LEVEL 4, ABSOLUTIST and LEVEL 6, SOCIOCENTRIC. Keep in mind, you are a combination of both. You are able to take the best of both. One does not compromise the other.

Self Motivation

Your brain activates in both the left and front. Skill improvement is best when you follow a two-phase process. First, you master the basics. This is done by focusing on proper positioning of your body and execution of the ideal, traditional muscle movement, i.e., proper stance and proper body movement. Once you master the basics without having to think, you move to the second phase, which is all mental. Here you focus on training your brain to feel the rhythm. Before execution, you first imagine what it feels like to execute perfectly. This feeling of what it is like to be a champion builds confidence. Confidence is knowing you are good. People who become very good at a skill develop an Olympian focus. For you, you first work the left side of the brain, mastering the basics, then you activate the front of the brain through visualizing what it feels like to execute perfectly. To get a better grasp of the procedure, read and master the Self Motivation section on LEVEL 4, ABSOLUTIST, then proceed to LEVEL 6, SOCIOCENTRIC. You are going to move from practice makes perfect to feeling perfection.

Strengths

Reliable; sensitive; self-disciplined; purposeful intentions

Weaknesses

Resistant to change; indecisive at times; worrisome; lack direction at times

Improvement

Become more visionary; master a physical skill; try out new things; become proactive

EPILOGUE

EPILOGUE

I have dedicated a substantial portion of my life to studying, researching, applying, and developing **PeopleWise® Motivation: The Art of Motivating Brain-to-Brain**. To me, **PeopleWise® Motivation** is more than a book or theory. It is more than a set of methods, techniques, or tricks. I believe it is the future and, for a select few, can be used to create the future through post-living.

It has affected my thinking and altered my behavior. Rather than evolving or unfolding, **PeopleWise® Motivation** develops through jerks and abrupt twists that form mind bursts. These mind bursts are insights, ah-hahs, paradigm shifts, breakthroughs that we refer to as "cows." The cow was shared with me by an employee from Hewlett Packard, as explained in Chapter 3. The photo of the cow originated in an article by K. M. Dallenbach (1951) found in the *American Journal of Psychology, Volume 64.*

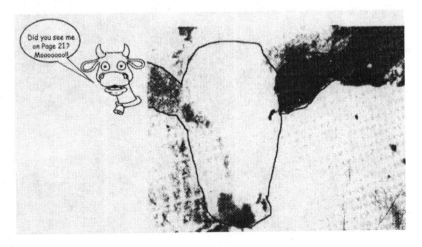

For me, **PeopleWise® Motivation** is a "cow" that is becoming more and more clear. **PeopleWise® Motivation** is too important to keep a secret, it is too important to keep to ourselves. Please share your **PeopleWise®** "cows" with me. All comments, suggestions, questions, and ideas are welcome.

James S. Payne
Management & Motivation, Inc.
P.O. Box 215
University, MS 38677
(662) 234-8846
mm@watervalley.net
FAX #: (662) 281-8780

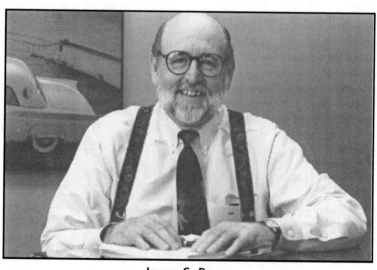

James S. Payne
President, Management & Motivation, Inc.

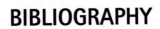

BIBLIOGRAPHY

BIBLIOGRAPHY

Armor, T. D. (1953). *How to play your best golf all the time.* New York: Simon & Schuster.

Blake, R. R., & Mouton, J. S. (1985). *The managerial grid III.* Houston: Gulf Publishing Company.

Block, J. R., & Yuker, H. E. (1989). *Can you believe your eyes?* New York: Gardner Press.

Block, P. (1987). *The empowered manager.* San Francisco: Jossey-Bass.

Brodsky, S. (1977). The mental health professional on the witness stand. In B. D. Sales (Ed.), *Psychology in the legal process.* New York: Spectrum Publishing.

Clark, G. (1973). *The man who tapped the secrets of the universe.* Waynesboro, VA: The University of Science and Philosophy.

Coffee, G. (1990). *Beyond survival.* Aiea, Hawaii: Coffee Enterprises.

Csikszentmihalyi, M. (1998). *Finding flow: The psychology of engagement with everyday life.* New York: HarperCollins.

Dallenbach, K. M. (1951). A puzzle-picture with a new principle of concealment. *American Journal of Psychology, 64,* 431–433.

Deming, W. E. (1986). *Out of the crisis.* Cambridge, MA: MIT Center for Advanced Engineering Study.

Deming, W. E. (1993). *The new economics.* Cambridge, MA: MIT Center for Advanced Engineering Study.

Diamond, M., & Hopson, J. (1998). *Magic trees of the mind: How to nuture your child's intelligence, creativity, and healthy emotions from birth through adolescence.* New York: Penguin Putnam.

Dyer, W. (1980). *The sky's the limit.* New York: Simon & Schuster.

Frankl, V. E. (1959). *Man's search for meaning.* New York: Simon & Schuster.

Gayle, W. (1959). *Power selling.* Englewood Cliffs, NJ: Prentice-Hall.

Glover, D. (1998). *Math like you've never seen it before* (videotape). Pittsburgh: WQED.

Goleman, D. (1995). *Emotional intelligence: Why it can matter more than I.Q.* New York: Bantam.

Graves, C. W. (1996). The deterioration of work standards. *Harvard Business Review, 44*, 117-126.

Graves, C. W. (1970). Levels of existence: An open system theory of values. *Journal of Humanistic Psychology, 10*, 131-155.

Graves, C. W. (1974). Human nature prepares for a momentous leap. *The Futurist, 8*, 72-87.

Hershey, G. L., & Lugo, J. O. (1970). *Living psychology.* London: Macmillan Company.

Kohlberg, L. (1984). *The psychology of moral development.* San Francisco: Harper and Row.

Kotulak, R. (1996). *Inside the brain: Revolutionary discoveries of how the mind works.* Kansas City, MO: Andrews & McMeely.

LeDoux, J. (1996). *The emotional brain: The mysterious underpinnings of emotional life.* New York: Simon & Schuster.

Maltz, M. (1967). *Psycho-cybernetics.* New York: Prentice Hall.

Maslow, A. H. (1971). *Toward a psychology of being.* Princeton, NJ: Van Nostrand.

Maslow, A. H. (1971). *The farther reaches of human nature.* New York: Viking Press.

Mayer, W. E. (1957). *Brainwashing . . . The ultimate weapon* (audio tape and transcription, source unknown).

McGregor, D. (1960). *The human side of enterprise.* New York: McGraw-Hill.

Myers, I. B. (1980). *Gifts differing.* Palo Alto: Consulting Psychologists Press.

Payne, J., Mercer, C., Payne, R., & Davison, R. (1973). *Head Start: A tragicomedy with epilogue.* New York: Behavioral Publications.

Payne, J., Polloway, E.,Kauffman, J., & Scranton, T. (1975). *Living in the classroom: The currency-based token economy.* New York: Human Sciences Press.

Peck, M. S. (1999). *Golf and the spirit.* New York: Harmony Books.

Peters, T. J. (1987). *Thriving on chaos.* New York: Alfred A. Knopf.

Polloway, E., Patton, J., Payne, J., & Payne, R. (1989). *Strategies for teaching learners with special needs* (4th ed.). New York: Merrill Publishing.

Tice, L. E. (1989). *A better world, a better you.* New jersey: Prentice Hall.

Thor, V. (1939). *Outwitting tomorrow.* La Miranda, CA: The Hover Company.

Waitley, D. (1983). *Seeds of greatness.* New York: Pocket Books.

ABOUT THE AUTHOR

James S. Payne is a recently-awarded Fulbright Scholar and presently serves as professor of Special Education at The University of Mississippi. He served as the Dean of the School of Education from 1985 to 1996. Prior to being a dean, he was a faculty member for 15 years at The University of Virginia. He received his doctorate, with honors, from The University of Kansas in 1970.

Dr. Payne has authored and coauthored numerous articles in professional journals and over 15 books, several of which were the largest-selling texts in their respective areas. *Mental Retardation: Introduction and Personal Perspectives* was the largest-selling introductory text in the area of mental retardation for over 14 years. *Strategies for Teaching the Mentally Retarded* was the largest selling methods text in the area of mental retardation for 12 years. *Exceptional Children in Focus* was the largest selling supplementary text in Special Education for 12 years. In 1990, Dr. Payne turned the authorship of the three texts over to students and colleagues so he could focus on his writing for the general public, mainly business and industry. The three texts remain best sellers under his mentorship and all are in their 6th and 7th editions. In 1994, Dr. Payne self-published *Differential Management and Motivation: An Advanced Understanding of Human Development and Motivation.* This was followed by *Differential Selling: A Primer.* For the past five years, his efforts have been directed toward developing the PeopleWise® system, of which *PeopleWise® Motivation: The Art of Motivating Brain-to-Brain* is an integral part. In 2001, Dr. Payne was granted the official trademark for PeopleWise® from the United States Patent Office. As part of the PeopleWise® system, Dr. Payne has developed *The PeopleWise® Event Management System*, which is a superior time management program, and The PeopleWise® Profile System, which is a self-scoring instrument that helps individuals understand themselves and others.

Dr. Payne is a nationally recognized speaker and trainer. He has appeared on numerous radio talk shows in 8 states, and presents regularly as a National Speakers Association professional speaker to more than 10,000 people a year.

Dr. Payne has consulted with both large and small organizations, such as South Central Bell; Federal Express; Dover Elevators; Washington Redskins; Caterpillar; City Government of Beverly Hills; City Government of Thornton, Colorado; Mercy Hospitals; HealthSouth; North Mississippi Medical Center; Virginia Power; Keesler Air Force Base; Franklin's Collection Services; Butner Federal Correctional Institute; Cary Hilliard Restaurants; Electrolux; Sto Corporation; Dunn-Edward Corporation; People's Bank; Federal Reserve Bank; and Pentagon Federal Credit Union. He has been a regular consultant with the Senior Executive Institute, teaching city managers team building and strategic planning, and the Federal Executive Institute, teaching federal executives vision building and motivation. Also, he has assisted salespersons with prospecting, qualifying, closing, and follow-up; athletes with attitude adjustment, physical training, and performance; attorneys on influence and persuasion techniques; and corporate executives in areas ranging from weight loss and divorce to decision making and delegation of authority.

In addition to being a university professor, he has been a paper boy, dishwasher, fry cook, iron foundry worker, farm hand, paint store clerk, oil-field worker, semi-pro baseball player, used-car salesperson, school teacher, and rehabilitation counselor. Administratively, he has been a restaurant manager, furniture stripping and repair proprietor, general manager of an automobile dealership, director of an early childhood education program, dean of a school of education and, presently, president of Management and Motivation, Inc.

Dr. Payne is the proud father of Kim and Janet. He was married for 38 consecutive years to Ruth Ann, who unfortunately passed away due to cancer in 1999. Dr. Payne recently married Esim, a university colleague. Esim originated from Turkey and has two sons, Burak and Firat. Jim and Esim currently reside in Oxford, Mississippi.